Stroke

Praise for *Stroke*

'Dr Aggarwal chose to write a book about stroke for the public. She faced a formidable task, summarizing information about a very complex topic that has been written about and studied for centuries. She has succeeded brilliantly. Writing in an easy-to-read, conversational style, she has brought to life key individuals, events and ideas about stroke. This book will undoubtedly stimulate readers to explore more about particular people and conditions and treatments.'

—**Louis R. Caplan, MD, Professor Emeritus,
Harvard Medical School, Boston**

'I read with great pleasure Dr Aggarwal's book discussing the medical history of stroke. She uses humour, anecdotes, science and a touch of humanity to describe the evolution of this field. It should be required reading for all future stroke doctors.'

—**Brian Jankowitz, MD, Chief of Neurosurgery,
JFK Neuroscience Institute, Edison**

'Stroke, often referred to as a brain attack, is a leading cause of disability and death worldwide. Alarmingly, more than two-thirds of strokes occur in low- and middle-income countries where there is a significant lack of awareness about stroke warning symptoms and signs among the general public.

'In *Stroke: A Medical History*, Dr Aishwarya Aggarwal delves into the fascinating and complex world of stroke, exploring its historical context, medical advancements and the profound impact it has on patients and their families. Dr Aggarwal provides an in-depth analysis of the causes of stroke, its treatment and prevention strategies, alongside a historical perspective.

'Through a compelling narrative and thorough research, this book offers a comprehensive understanding of the history of stroke for the general public and for anyone interested in the evolution of stroke medicine. Congratulations to Dr Aggarwal for this fabulous work.'

—Jeyaraj Durai Pandian, MD, Professor of Neurology; Principal, Christian Medical College, Ludhiana; and President, World Stroke Organization

'*Stroke: A Medical History* is a prodigious work by Dr Aishwarya Aggarwal. History buffs, the general public and even seasoned medical professionals alike will find this book a treasure trove. Dr Aggarwal has painstakingly researched and brought to light the astonishing ways in which the science of stroke care has evolved—from the time of Hippocrates to the modern era—not through logical steps or the work of large groups, but in fits and starts, driven by dedicated scientists and physicians singularly focused on uncovering the mysteries of this devastating disease and finding ways to overcome it.

'Even for stroke experts like me, the chapter on clot busters held a complete surprise: the discovery of streptokinase was serendipitously based on the study of antibiotics and the acute observation of their effects, rather than on the deliberate design of an agent or chemical to dissolve clots. Such nuggets and pearls of insight fill every paragraph of this remarkable book, making it an enjoyable read at every level.'

—Dileep R. Yavagal, MD, Professor of Clinical Neurology and Neurosurgery, University of Miami, Miami

Stroke

A Medical History

AISHWARYA AGGARWAL

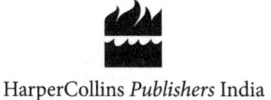

HarperCollins *Publishers* India

First published in India by HarperCollins *Publishers* 2025
4th Floor, Tower A, Building No. 10, DLF Cyber City,
DLF Phase II, Gurugram, Haryana – 122002
www.harpercollins.co.in

2 4 6 8 10 9 7 5 3 1

Copyright © Aishwarya Aggarwal 2025
Illustrations in 'Introduction' and 'Thunderclap' © Aishwarya Aggarwal 2025
Illustration in 'Blood Thinners' © Joe D/Wikimedia
Commons/CC-BY-SA-3.0/GFDLv1.2
Photograph in 'World History and Stroke' © National Archives (NAID: 531340)

P-ISBN: 978-93-6569-885-5
E-ISBN: 978-93-6569-882-4

The views and opinions expressed in this book are the author's own and the facts are as reported by her, and the publishers are not in any way liable for the same. None of the content in this book is intended to be a substitute for professional medical advice and should not be relied on as health or medical advice, diagnosis or treatment. Always seek the guidance of your doctor or other qualified health professional with any questions you may have regarding your health or a medical condition.

Aishwarya Aggarwal asserts the moral right
to be identified as the author of this work.

All rights reserved. No part of this publication may be reproduced, stored in a retrieval system, or transmitted, in any form or by any means, electronic, mechanical, photocopying, recording or otherwise, without the prior permission of the publishers.

Typeset in 12/16 Adobe Garamond Pro at
HarperCollins *Publishers* India

Printed and bound at
Thomson Press (India) Ltd.

This book is produced from independently certified FSC® paper
to ensure responsible forest management.

A tribute to the work, writings and teachings of my professor and mentor, Dr Louis R. Caplan

and

to my pillars of strength, my parents, Dr Saroj Aggarwal and Dr Anil Aggarwal

CONTENTS

	Author's Note	xi
	Introduction	xv
1.	The Circle of Willis	1
2.	On the Motion of the Heart and Blood	12
3.	Virchow's Triad	22
4.	The Heart and Brain Connection	30
5.	No-Man's Land	46
6.	Blood Thinners	55
7.	Clot Busters and Retrievers	71
8.	Imaging	86
9.	Thunderclap	112
10.	'Time Is Brain'	125
11.	Abilities versus Disabilities	134
12.	Stroke in the Young	151
13.	Genes	164
14.	Prevention Is Better than Cure	172
15.	World History and Stroke	187
	Acknowledgements	199
	References	205
	Index	235

Author's Note

MY JOURNEY INTO the world of stroke began as a medical student at Christian Medical College, Ludhiana. Here, under the guidance of Dr Jeyaraj Pandian, I encountered stroke patients for the first time and witnessed their treatment and management. In August 2019, as a final-year medical student, I embarked on a transformative three-month clinical elective at Harvard Medical School. The Longwood Medical Area, home to iconic institutions like Harvard Medical School and Boston Children's Hospital, felt like sacred ground. This stint at Harvard brought me to the very place where prominent historical medical figures like the renowned neurosurgeon Harvey Cushing had once worked.

Serendipity, an unexpected yet fortunate discovery, often accompanies remarkable inventions and findings. While crafting this book, I experienced my own serendipitous moment. During the second week of my rotation, I found a neurology note penned by Dr Louis R. Caplan while reviewing a patient's charts. Having read Dr Caplan's books, I was thrilled to learn that this esteemed stroke expert was still practising at Beth Israel Deaconess Medical Center at the age of eighty-two! Mustering courage, I visited the neurology clinic the next day, rehearsing my introduction while waiting outside his office as he attended to a patient. To my surprise, Dr Caplan turned out to be one of the kindest individuals I would meet, eventually becoming my mentor. Meeting him affirmed my belief that the universe supported my mission to write about stroke.

Currently, as a neurology resident, caring for stroke patients has further deepened my commitment to this field. Each encounter with a patient reinforces my passion and dedication to understanding and treating stroke, shaping my journey in this profound and impactful specialty.

I don't want to lose you, my readers, after the first two chapters by making this book a detailed history lesson. Instead, with this book, I've made an attempt to take you on a journey through experiences that engage and enlighten. We'll celebrate the giants who paved the way for us in medicine and gain inspiration from their stories. I'll also be sharing my personal experiences, including lessons learnt from being in medicine, and those that I've gleaned from my mentors and my patients.

While I've attempted to cover some of the most significant developments in the field of medicine, this book is in no way a definitive chronicle. The history of developments in the field of stroke medicine spans centuries and multiple disciplines, making it near impossible to give a detailed account of it all in a book of this length. What I offer is an insight into the nature of the disease and an overview of the evolution of concepts, diagnostic

AUTHOR'S NOTE

techniques and treatments pertaining to stroke. This work rests heavily on the shoulders of countless research papers, books, articles and interviews published over the last century, and for these I am indebted.

—Dr Aishwarya Aggarwal

Introduction

*The farther backward you can look, the farther forward
you can see.*

—Winston Churchill

*We are like dwarfs sitting on the shoulders of giants.
We see more, and things that are more distant, than they did,
not because our sight is superior or because we are taller than
they, but because they raise us up, and by their great stature
add to ours.*

—John of Salisbury

OVER 2,400 YEARS ago, Hippocrates (c. 460–c. 370 BCE), hailed as the father of medicine, was the first to recognize what we know today as a stroke. He used the term 'apoplexy', Greek for 'struck down by violence'. The term was employed by the Greeks because of its catastrophic presentation: a sudden loss of consciousness, motion and sensation. Hippocrates noted that apoplexy was most common among those between forty and sixty years of age, and he described it as a patient experiencing sudden pain and a loss of speech, accompanied with a rattle in the throat, urinating without awareness and being unresponsive. He further stated that, 'It is impossible to remove a strong attack of apoplexy, and not easy to remove a weak attack.'

According to Hippocrates, the pathogenesis of apoplexy was linked to the humoral theory. The four humours of Hippocratic medicine are black bile, yellow bile, phlegm and blood. It was believed that these four humours must be in balanced proportions with regards to amount and potency for a body to be healthy. This equilibrium was known as 'eukrasia' (a normal state of health). An imbalance or separation of the humours was thought to result in diseases.

In the era of Hippocrates and even Galen (130–210 CE), physicians had little knowledge of the anatomy and function of the brain. Hippocrates believed that blood held our spirit, or 'vitality', and any interference with the flow of vitality to the brain would result in apoplexy. His hypothesis was supported by his proponent Galen, who also believed that apoplexy arose from imbalances in the humours, such as an accumulation of phlegm or black bile in the cerebral ventricles. Galen's theory held sway until the seventeenth century, when physicians began dissecting human bodies.

Johann Jakob Wepfer (1620–95) is credited with being the first to observe apoplexy's correlation with cerebral haemorrhages (bleeding in the brain). In his examinations of cadavers, he demonstrated the absence of black bile or phlegm in the cerebral ventricles of those who had died of apoplexy, thus challenging Galen's theory.

Today, 'apoplexy' is no longer a familiar medical term, supplanted in clinical practice by 'stroke'. The etymology of the word goes back to historical perceptions. According to medical historian Francis Schiller, the first synonym for 'stroke of the palsy' in the 1599 edition of the Oxford English Dictionary was 'stroke of God's hands'. The term implied that the condition was caused by an act of divine intervention; the patient appeared to be struck by lightning, or by the hand of God.

Before we delve deeper into the history of stroke, let us briefly review our current understanding of the condition.

Annually, over thirteen million people worldwide have a stroke, with around five and a half million dying as a result. Globally, there are over eighty million people who have experienced a stroke at least once. Stroke is a leading cause of death and disability, with over 116 million years of healthy life lost each year.

What exactly is a stroke? The term is used to describe a brain injury caused by an abnormality in the blood supply to a part of the brain. Most stroke patients are stricken suddenly by the blood vessel abnormality, and abnormalities of brain function can also begin quickly, sometimes within an instant. When a part of the brain does not receive adequate oxygen and glucose due to insufficient blood supply to that area, it fails to function. For instance, if a vessel supplying blood to the part of the brain that controls speech is blocked, the patient will present with a loss of speech.

Strokes can be divided into two very broad groups: haemorrhage and ischemia. Haemorrhage, named for the Greek *haima*, meaning 'blood' and *rhegnunai*, meaning 'to break forth';

a free and forceful escape of blood, refers to bleeding inside the skull, either within the brain or in the fluid surrounding the brain. Ischemia, which gets its name from the Greek *iskhaimos*, meaning 'to hold back blood', refers to a lack of blood flow to the brain. Brain ischemia is much more common than haemorrhages—around four out of every five strokes are ischemic.

To grasp this better, imagine a river carrying water to a stretch of land, the river being its only source of water. Analogous to ischemia would be the river running dry before reaching the land. It could be due to say a dam built on it somewhere on its way, preventing further flow of water or its source drying up. If the area were to be deprived of water for too long, all its vegetation would eventually die. In the context of the brain, a vessel is usually blocked due to a blood clot that forms within the vessel or travels from a distant site. Ischemia in the brain could result from a general low blood pressure state in the body which can arise due to excessive blood loss, from bleeding, or dehydration. It could also be due to a problem with the heart (the pump), leading to a diminished blood flow to the head and the brain.

It has been estimated that a patient loses 1.9 million neurons in the brain each minute it is deprived of its blood supply. Thus, the phrase 'time is brain' emphasizes that the human nervous system faces rapid, irreversible damage as a stroke progresses, necessitating urgent treatment.

If the river drying up is ischemia, a haemorrhage is the opposite—it's a tsunami. Much like how floods destroy structures, bleeding in the brain disconnects vital nerve centres and pathways. A haemorrhage usually results from the rupture of small blood vessels within the brain substance, most commonly due to very high blood pressure. The blood oozes into the brain under pressure and forms a localized mass, often round or elliptical, called a haematoma. Haematomas also exert pressure on the brain regions adjacent to the collected blood and can injure these neuronal structures as well. Given the skull's constrained space, very large haemorrhages can often be fatal because they increase pressure within the skull, squeezing vital parts of the brainstem, such as the region that controls breathing.

The heart pumps the blood to the rest of the body through the aorta, the largest artery in the body. The aorta divides into some main branches including those that supply the brain and pass through the neck. The blood from the brain re-enters the heart through the veins. Any abnormality within this continuous loop—from the heart to the aorta, to the neck arteries, to the brain arteries and, finally, back through the veins to the heart—can cause a stroke.

The first branch arising from the right side of the aorta is the brachiocephalic trunk, or the innominate artery. This vessel then branches into the right subclavian artery and the right common carotid artery. The right subclavian artery, which runs under the clavicle to supply blood to the right arm, also gives rise to the right vertebral artery, which supplies blood to the lower back portion of the right side of the brain. Meanwhile, the right common carotid artery further bifurcates, with the right external carotid artery serving the right side of the face and neck, and the right internal carotid artery supplying blood to the front of the right half of the brain and the right eye.

Coming back to the aorta, the next branch is the left common carotid artery. This branches into the left external carotid artery, catering to the left side of the face and neck, and the left internal carotid artery, which supplies the front of the left half of the brain and the left eye.

The last branch of the aorta is the left subclavian artery. This gives rise to the left vertebral artery, which supplies blood to the lower back portion of the left side of the brain. Both the left and the right vertebral arteries join to form the basilar artery, tasked with supplying blood to the rest of the back portion of the brain (see figures 1 and 2).

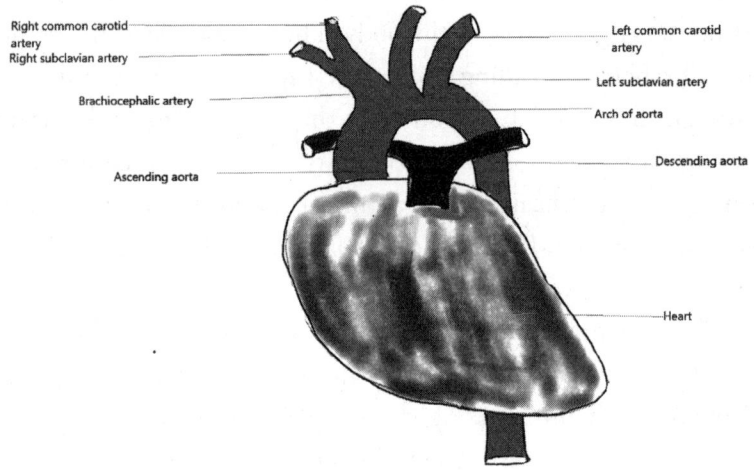

Figure 1 Branches of the aorta

Inside the skull, each internal carotid artery divides into the middle cerebral artery, which mainly supplies the structures on the outer lateral surface of the cerebral hemispheres, and the anterior cerebral artery, which supplies the brain structures near the midline. The back of the cerebral hemispheres is supplied by the posterior cerebral arteries, which branch from the basilar artery (see figure 3).

INTRODUCTION xxi

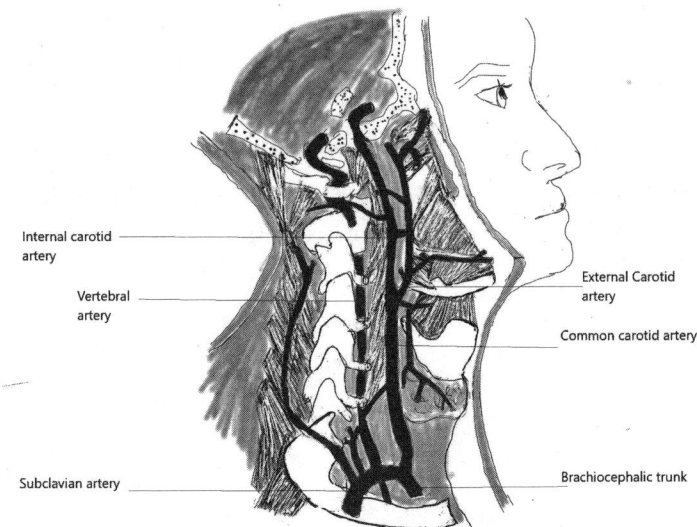

Figure 2 Arteries on the right side of the neck

The arteries supplying the frontal portions of the brain connect with those supplying the posterior portions. Additionally, the

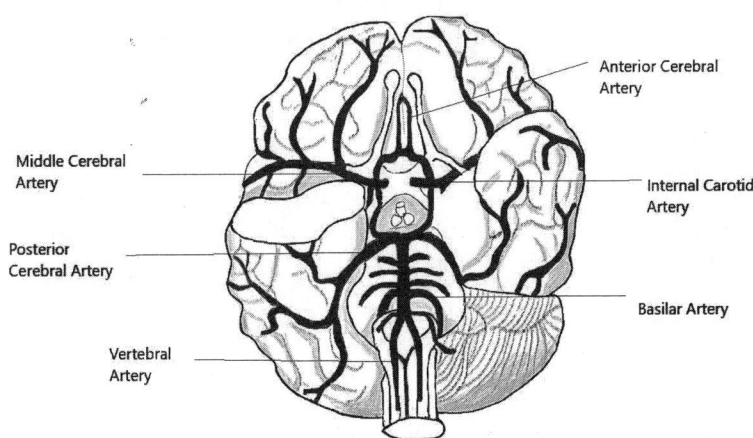

Figure 3 Arteries supplying the brain

arteries from the brain's left side join those from its right side. This joining of the arteries is called the Circle of Willis. Comprising this 'circle' are the two anterior cerebral arteries, connected by the anterior communicating artery, the two internal carotid arteries and the two posterior cerebral arteries, which are joined together by the posterior communicating arteries (see figure 4).

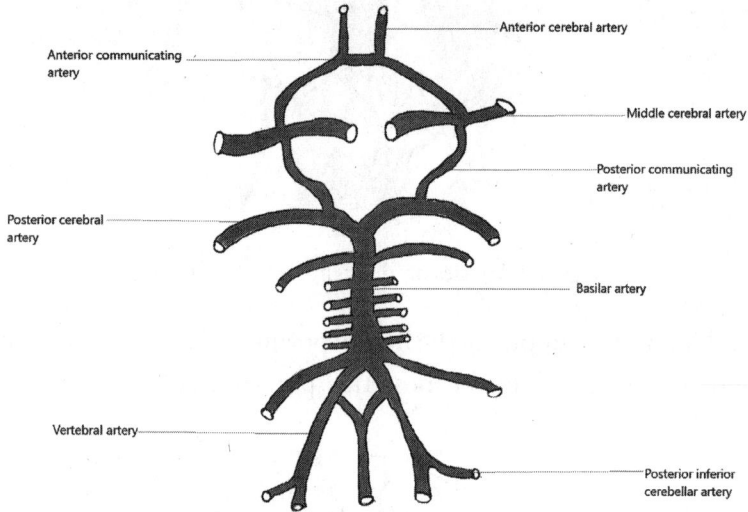

Figure 4 The Circle of Willis

1

The Circle of Willis

If you find from your own experience that something is a fact and it contradicts what some authority has written down, then you must abandon the authority and base your reasoning on your own findings.

—Leonardo da Vinci

HEROPHILUS OF CHALCEDON (335–280 BCE) was the first to perform human dissections. He dissected more than 600 human cadavers in his lifetime. One of his profound observations was the intricate vascular structure at the base of the brain, which he termed *rete mirabile*, meaning 'wonderful net'. Sadly, much of his work was destroyed during Julius Caesar's invasion of Alexandria. Yet, it is believed that Galen preserved and incorporated some of Herophilus's findings into his own teachings.

Galen of Pergamon, a Greek physician, surgeon and philosopher in the Roman Empire, is considered one of the most accomplished medical researchers of antiquity. He influenced the development of various scientific disciplines, including anatomy, physiology, pathology, pharmacology and neurology. In the ninth volume of his *De Usu Partium Corporis Humani* (*On the Usefulness of the Parts of the Body*), he described the rete mirabile in detail. He extolled it as the most wonderful of the bodies, encircling the hypophysis (pituitary gland) and lying as a plexus at the base of the brain. He likened it to several fishing nets layered upon each other, each layer being tightly attached to and inseparable from the next. Beyond its structure, Galen theorized its physiological role. According to him, chyle from the digestive tract was transformed in the liver into a 'natural pneuma' or 'spirit'. In the heart, pneuma, prepared from air inhaled by the lungs, combined with this natural spirit to form the 'vital spirit'. The vital spirit then travelled up the carotid arteries into the rete mirabile in the brain, where it was transformed into the 'animal' or 'psychic' pneuma. The tortuous structure of the rete mirabile slowed down the blood flow, allowing this transformation. The animal spirit was considered the highest form of spirit as it was distributed through the nerves and provided sensation and empowered motion.

However, a significant revelation disrupts Galen's detailed account. The rete mirabile that Galen described does not exist in humans. Galen's anatomical descriptions were based on animal dissections, as human dissections were forbidden by the Church in his time. He learnt about the human anatomy from treating wounded gladiators and by performing surgeries, but never through human dissections. His primary subjects for dissection were apes and ungulates, and in one of his books, he states that a particular description is that of an ox. Despite this, Galen's teaching prevailed unchallenged for centuries.

૭

Andreas Vesalius was born on 31 December 1514 in Brussels, Belgium. His father, an apothecary, catered to the Habsburg family. Many in his family were scholars or physicians, some also serving royalty. The family library was extensive, and as a boy, Vesalius developed a keen reading habit. At fifteen, he left Brussels to study at the University of Louvain, where he was taught Latin, Greek, philosophy, rhetoric and some Hebrew, eventually earning a Master of Arts degree.

Vesalius had decided on a medical career, but since Louvain did not have an outstanding medical school, at eighteen, he travelled to Paris. There, he found himself immersed in the writings of Galen. He conducted his first human cadaveric dissection in Paris and became fascinated by anatomy. During his third year of study, however, war beset France, so Vesalius returned to Belgium and finished his medical studies at the University of Louvain, earning a Bachelor of Medicine degree. His medical studies then took him to Padua, where he underwent bedside training. In December 1537, he was granted a Doctor of Medicine degree with distinction. The day after his graduation, he was appointed professor of surgery and anatomy.

On his first day as a professor, Vesalius began a series of cadaveric dissections that revolutionized traditional anatomy lessons. Before him, lecturers would sit on a high chair in front of the students and read aloud Galenic texts in Latin while assistants performed dissections that the lecturer could not even see. The primary purpose of these sessions was to reaffirm Galenic teachings. Instead of being removed from the action, Vesalius merged the roles of surgeon, lecturer and demonstrator. He displayed a skeleton near the dissection table for the students' reference and then began by sketching an outline of the bones on the cadaver's skin. His teachings were supplemented by large anatomical charts, dissections and even vivisections of small animals to demonstrate living organs or comparative anatomy. His innovative lectures attracted large audiences of both students and colleagues.

During a public dissection, Vesalius dissected the brain of a sheep, showcasing the three ventricles and the rete mirabile. In the following years, he dissected many human cadavers, usually executed criminals, and compiled his findings in his prodigious book *De Humani Corporis Fabrica,* published in 1543. The Canadian physician William Osler extolled it as the greatest book ever written, and historians ranked it first among the ten greatest medical discoveries. The late historian Roy Porter has described it as 'one of the pearls of Renaissance printing'.

Vesalius started as a Galenic anatomist and followed his advice of 'seeing for oneself'. However, as he became adept in human dissection, he concluded that Galen's teachings were entirely based on animal dissections. In his book, Vesalius corrected some 200 anatomical errors made by Galen. At the time, it was bold of Vesalius to challenge Galen's teachings. As he noted:

> How much has been attributed to Galen, easily leader of the professors of dissection, by those physicians and anatomists who have followed him, and often against reason! ... Indeed, I myself cannot wonder enough at my own stupidity and too

great trust in the writings of Galen and other anatomists; yes I, who so much laboured in my love for Galen that I never undertook to dissect a human head in public without that of a lamb or ox at hand, so as to supply what I could in no way find in that of a man, and to impress it on the spectators, lest I be charged with failure to find that plexus so universally familiar by name. For the soporal [carotid] arteries quite fail to produce such a plexus reticularis as that which Galen recounts.

Though Vesalius did not describe the arterial circle as we know it today, his description was much closer to reality than the then-acclaimed rete mirabile.

Many improvements were made in the model of the vascular structure at the base of the brain described by Vesalius. Important contributions were made by eminent researchers like Gabriele Falloppio, Giulio Casserio, Johann Vesling and Johann Jakob Wepfer to the understanding of the arterial network.

The Invisible College, also known as the Philosophical College, was an informal group established by several scientifically minded people at Oxford. They met every Thursday to perform experiments and exchange knowledge. The group is regarded by many as the precursor to the Royal Society of London. Among the group were physician Thomas Willis, philosopher and physicist Robert Boyle, mathematician John Wallis, architect and anatomist Christopher Wren, economist and physician Sir William Petty, philosopher John Locke and physician Richard Lower.

Born on 27 January 1621 in Wiltshire, southwest of London, Thomas Willis was the oldest among three sons and three daughters. The siblings lost their mother when Thomas was just ten. Every day, he walked two miles to and from Sylvester's Academy, a local private school known for its classical education in Latin and Greek. At sixteen, Willis matriculated at the University of Oxford as a servitor to Dr Thomas Iles, a canon of Christ Church. Servitors were usually bright youngsters from humble circumstances who performed menial tasks in exchange for free housing and tuition. Mrs Iles, though not a trained physician, practised medicine and surgery, and was known to cure patients of various ailments. Willis spent significant time under her guidance. He graduated with a Bachelor of Arts degree in 1639, and three years later, earned a Master of Arts degree.

Thomas initially intended to be ordained as an Anglican clergyman. His entry into medicine was attributable to an accident of times. During a civil war that began shortly after he graduated, a severe epidemic, possibly typhus, led to the deaths of his father and stepmother. His ecclesiastical aspirations came to a halt as he returned home, now responsible for managing two farms and parenting and educating his younger siblings. In 1646, half a year after the civil war ended, Willis received his medical education as a reward for his loyalty to the Crown. That same year, Oxford relinquished to the parliamentary forces, due to which Willis's course was cut short. He did not have to undergo the traditional Oxford medical training of studying the works of Aristotle, Hippocrates and Galen. This proved advantageous, freeing Willis from entrenched misconceptions and allowing him to conduct his own experiments instead.

Studying the anatomy of the brain was a difficult task then, for the organ decayed fast and the prevalent approach to its dissection had several limitations. Traditional anatomists did not extract the brain as a whole but dissected it in slices after opening the vault. Willis, along with his colleagues from the Invisible College, removed the intact brain from the vault, which significantly improved their study of its vascular structure.

Robert Boyle, renowned for his discovery of showing that the volume of a gas is inversely proportional to its pressure (commonly known as Boyle's Law), made a significant contribution to anatomical studies by introducing the groundbreaking concept of preservation. He suggested the use of alcohol for the preservation of the human body after he noticed that wine prevented fish from rotting. This technique was adopted by Willis and his colleagues for the preservation of the brain.

Along with Wren, Boyle began studying the effects of viper venom on dogs, utilizing the technique of intravenous injection invented by Wren. Willis used this technique to inject dye into the carotid arteries. As the dye flowed through the lumen of the blood vessels, it traced the entire vasculature of the brain and demonstrated the anastomosis or connections between the vessels that formed a circle.

With assistance from Richard Lower, an anatomist of tremendous dexterity and precision, Willis elucidated the anatomical structure of the brain. In 1664, he published his book *Cerebri Anatome: Cui Accessit Nervorum Descriptio et Usus* (*The Anatomy of the Brain and Nerves*). The precise and detailed illustration of the 'Circle of Willis' in this work was prepared by Christopher Wren, who later designed the iconic St. Paul's Cathedral in London.

Willis went a step further and tried to relate the anatomical structure to its function. He autopsied a man who had died of an abdominal tumour but was neurologically asymptomatic and reported his findings:

> When his skull was opened, we noted amongst the usual intracranial findings, the right carotid artery, in its intracranial part, bony or even hard, its lumen, being almost totally occluded; so that influx of blood being denied by this route, it seemed remarkable that this person had not died previously of an apoplexy. Nature has substituted a sufficient remedy against the danger of apoplexy; as the vertebral artery on the same side, in which the carotid was occluded, became thrice as big as both its pipes on the other side.

The man had not suffered from apoplexy despite the fact that his right carotid artery was totally blocked. This was because the right vertebral artery grew in size and carried more blood, which was eventually redistributed from the back of the brain to the front through the circular connection between them.

In order to confirm his findings, Willis conducted an experiment with Wren. They tied both the carotid arteries of a spaniel and found the dog to be completely asymptomatic. Later, when they examined the inside of its head, they found that all the vessels were engorged with blood. The blood had been provided by the vertebral arteries through the Circle of Willis.

We were a batch of seventy-five medical students at Christian Medical College, Ludhiana. The first year of our medical curriculum included the study of the anatomy, physiology and biochemistry of the human body. Anatomy (*ana*, meaning 'up' and *temnein*, meaning 'to cut') is the study of the structure of the human body. Physiology (*physis*, meaning 'nature, origin' and *logia*, meaning 'study of') is the study of the functions and mechanisms of a living system. Biochemistry is the study of chemical processes within and relating to living organisms.

On our second day of med school, we were taken to the dissection hall, or, as we called it, the D-Hall. Laid before us were five cadavers, each draped in a white sheet and designated for a group of fifteen students. Over the following year, we were to dissect the cadaver assigned to us part by part. A cadaver is a distinct educational tool, as it is neither the student's 'first patient' nor a mere biological model. It cannot be harmed by the student and its use is ethically sound.

Our extended dissection period of a whole year was made possible through the preservation of the cadavers via embalming, further aided by refrigeration. Embalming is the art and science of preserving human remains by treating them with chemicals to forestall decomposition. The most commonly used fluid is concentrated formaldehyde, known as formalin. Since embalming is done through the circulatory system, the fluid is injected into an artery under high pressure and flow, and is then allowed to swell and saturate the tissues. After the cadaver is left to sit for a number of hours, the venous system is generally opened to let the fluid drain. As the formaldehyde mixes with the blood, it gives a grey hue to the cadavers, known as formaldehyde grey or embalmer's grey.

Upon our first encounter with the cadavers, a few students, hit by the stench of the formalin, came close to swooning, and some left the hall to puke. But it wasn't long before we all got used to the smell of formalin and dissection in D-Hall. We were instructed to treat the cadavers with respect and to pay tribute to their souls. Students were almost never haunted by the idea of working on a dead body. We were also issued a set of seven or eight human bones to study in detail, and around exam time, many students often slept with the set at their bedside.

My fondest memory of D-Hall is when my dissection partner and I meticulously exposed the abdominal blood vessels supplying the stomach and the intestines. Those were the two most gruelling hours of dissection for me. Carefully removing the fascia and fat that covered the arteries, separating them from adjacent veins and nerves, we slowly unveiled a beautiful network of arteries: large ones connected to each other and smaller branches covering the gut like a woven net. I was in awe of its sheer artistry. Perhaps it was experiences like these that drove pioneer anatomists like Vesalius to actually steal the corpses of executed criminals for dissection.

Today, we are fortunate to learn anatomy with the aid of well-preserved and prepared cadavers, virtual simulators and digital resources. Platforms like Google give us instant access to information and pictures, and cameras document our findings. Vesalius and Willis had to employ artists to illustrate their dissections. Before the evolution of printing techniques in the 1800s, most anatomy atlases were hand-drawn, limiting the spread of this knowledge.

Various printing techniques began to evolve around the turn of the nineteenth century. The printing techniques using traditional black ink included woodcut, cross-hatching, stipple engraving, mezzotint and aquatint. To add colour, different methods were employed. The simplest was to add colour by hand, and low-ranked artists were made to individually colour all the plates, usually not more than a few hundred. Early in the eighteenth century, Jacob Christoph Le Blon, inspired by Newton's colour theory, devised a multi-plate colour printing technique. Utilizing separate plates for red, blue and yellow, he later added a fourth plate for black. A different technique, called *à la poupée*, involved using only one plate to which different colours were strategically applied using a cloth or a paintbrush. An important advancement in printing was the development of lithography. Lithography was a planographic printing process that made use of the natural repulsion between grease and water.

The mid-nineteenth century witnessed a surge in knowledge dissemination related to the pathology of stroke, mainly through the publication of four prominent atlases by physicians Robert Hooper, Richard Bright, Jean Cruveilhier and Robert Carswell. Lithography was used in the work of Jean Cruveilhier and Robert Carswell. Published anatomy and pathology atlases helped physicians who did not perform autopsies to visualize the pathology in the brain. Atlases were a true example of the adage, 'a picture is worth a thousand words' in the visual advances they made.

2

On the Motion of the Heart and Blood

All we know is still infinitely less than that remains unknown.

—William Harvey

GALEN'S WRITINGS AND teachings dominated medical practice for about 1,500 years, remaining unchallenged until the sixteenth century. This was when Vesalius and Harvey brought to light the study of anatomy and physiology. Galen, a proponent of the humoral theory, believed blood to be the dominant humour and greatly promoted the practice of bloodletting as a means to restore humoral balance. Notably, Charles II (1630–85) underwent extensive bloodletting following a stroke. The practice persisted well into the twentieth century. In fact, the esteemed medical journal *The Lancet* derives its name from the lancet, a sharp, pointed, double-edged surgical instrument that was imperative to medical practice at the time. Physicians would carry lancets and fleams (an instrument used for bloodletting) in their pockets and would make cuts in their patients' veins to bleed them. Other methods included cupping and leech therapy. Rows of patients would stand outside hospitals waiting to be bled at their own request, for it was believed that bleeding every spring brought vigour.

However, the treatment of bloodletting was based on a major flaw in Galen's understanding of human physiology. Galen believed that there were two different types of blood, each with a distinct pathway. According to him, the venous blood was continuously produced in the liver from food and was absorbed by the tissues without ever returning to the heart. Arterial blood, on the other hand, originated in the heart and was the source of vitality, and, like venous blood, did not return to the heart.

The fact that blood flows in a circular motion in the body was not discovered until 1628. The discovery was so unexpected that its discoverer grappled with its implications, worried that challenging the teachings of Galen would jeopardize his medical practice.

William Harvey was born on 1 April 1578 in a coastal town in England. He hailed from a prosperous family and was the oldest of nine children. One of his brothers, Eliab, who became quite wealthy, managed William's monetary affairs, ensuring he never faced financial difficulties. He began his formal education at King's School in Canterbury, where students were required to communicate in only Latin or Greek. An ardent student of the classics throughout his life, he became fluent in both languages. At sixteen, he enrolled in Gonville and Caius College, Cambridge, an institution known for matriculating students interested in medicine. Each year there, the bodies of two executed criminals were dissected in the presence of students. Like the great anatomist Vesalius, Harvey enrolled in the University of Padua, Italy, at the age of nineteen in 1597, to attain his medical degree. He studied anatomy and physiology under Hieronymus Fabricius, who is credited with the discovery of venous valves but was unable to explain their function.

Harvey returned to London in 1602 and became a member of the Royal College of Physicians, for which he gave annual lectures on anatomy. He served as an attending physician at St. Bartholomew's Hospital and was one of the royal physicians to James I and, later, Charles I.

Harvey was Aristotelian in his beliefs and very ambitious. He was inclined to discover the secrets of nature by studying the structure of animal bodies. As he wrote, 'The examination of the bodies of animals has always been my delight; and I have thought that we might thence not only obtain insight into the ... mysteries of Nature, but there perceive a kind of image or reflex of the omnipotent Creator himself'. He also believed in conducting his own experiments as he said, 'I learn anatomy not from books but from dissections, not from the tenets of Philosophers but from the fabric of nature.'

Harvey, therefore, set out to find the structure, function and peculiarities of the hearts of as many animal species as he could find. He dissected over eighty different species, including fleas, deer, snakes, fish, rats, turtles, silkworms, dogs, cats, molluscs, sheep, bees and geese. All these were carried out in his wife's kitchen. Harvey was ruthless, unshaken by the shrieking of the live animals as he dissected them. When his wife's beloved parrot died, he dissected it too, and discovered that it wasn't a male as he had previously thought, but a female, who died due to a decaying egg in its oviduct.

In the rapidly beating hearts of most of the animals, it was impossible to discern if the auricles contracted before the ventricles. To overcome this problem, Harvey observed the hearts of cold-blooded animals, such as fish, which beat at a slower rate, and waited as warm-blooded animals died in front of him and their hearts become slower and slower. Through these experiments he concluded that the auricles contracted first and ejected the blood into the ventricles, which contracted later. Harvey thus proposed that the function of the heart was to pump blood to the extremities, and the force of the transmission was felt as pulsations in the arteries.

Harvey's approach was not limited to observation but was supplemented by his application of mathematics. By measuring the volume of blood in the left ventricle of a dog's heart and multiplying this by the number of heartbeats per minute, he determined that the left ventricle ejected about three pounds of blood in half an hour. This was almost equal to the total blood volume of the dog. It was not conceivable that such a large amount of blood could be replaced by the blood produced in the liver from chyle or that it could be continually absorbed by the tissues. Harvey thus concluded that the blood had to have a specific movement in the body: that it was pumped by the heart into the arteries, which carried it to the tissues, while the veins brought it back to the heart from the tissues. The motion was thus 'circular'.

He further substantiated the concept of circulation by occluding the single vein leading to the beating heart of a snake. The heart became pale, shrank and stopped ejecting blood into the aorta. On releasing the occlusion, the heart regained its colour and again pumped blood into the aorta. He also demonstrated that when a ligature was applied to a vein, the segment below it swelled while the segment above collapsed, indicating the direction of flow towards the heart. He also discerned the function of valves in veins—that they allow blood to flow only in one direction. This was confirmed by the fact that a probe could be passed in a vein only in one direction: the apparent direction of the flow of blood.

Anatomically, arteries are placed deeper in the body while veins are superficial. In one of Harvey's experiments, he applied a ligature on the arm of a human volunteer. The ligature was tight enough to occlude both the arteries and veins. This caused the arm to become pale, cold and painful, with the veins visible superficially collapsing. Upon slightly loosening the ligature so that it allowed arterial blood to flow but continued to occlude the vein, he observed that the arm and the hand regained their colour and became warm. The veins became distended with blood as the loosened ligature still prevented its further escape. This established that blood flowed from the arteries into the veins. However, Harvey could not observe the precise connections as the microscope was yet to be invented. It was Marcello Malpighi who, in 1661, used a microscope to detect capillaries, the tiny vessels that connect arteries to veins.

Harvey's discovery had the potential to upend Galen's physiology and the therapeutics based on it. Therefore, he cautiously garnered the support of his Royal College colleagues over nine years, presenting them with ocular demonstrations before publishing his work. His seminal work, *Exercitatio Anatomica de Motu Cordis et Sanguinis in Animalibus* (*On the Motion of the Heart and Blood*), was published in 1628 in Frankfurt. Despite his research, he faced criticism from his European contemporaries for his discovery. In 1657, William Harvey died of a stroke.

∽

I feel fortunate that by the time I began medical school, the University Grants Commission (the government body that regulates university education in India) had banned animal dissection. Largely due to its widespread use in dissections, the Indian bullfrog population declined drastically and became endangered. There is no need to sacrifice animals to demonstrate concepts that can be easily explained using computer software and simulators. So, I can admit that I have not seen the beating heart of a dying animal. Nevertheless, our curriculum had plenty of lectures devoted to the cardiovascular system—the heart and the blood vessels. Beyond its intricate structural design, the human body's functioning is just as marvellous. The ubiquitous laws of physics that govern our universe also apply to the human body.

To push blood throughout the body, the heart needs to overcome the resistance offered by the blood vessels, which is known as vascular resistance. The blood vessels don't have a constant diameter; they change in response to various conditions or stressors, and are controlled by chemicals and hormones in the blood. Vasoconstriction is when the diameter of a vessel decreases and offers more resistance to blood flow. Vasodilation is when the diameter of a vessel increases, enhancing blood flow. For example, during exercise, muscles demand more oxygen. The blood vessels will vasodilate to increase the amount of blood and, therefore, oxygen being delivered to those muscles.

The sympathetic nervous system and various hormones in the body control its overall vascular tone. But different organs, like the kidneys, lungs and brain, have their own mechanisms to control the amount of blood flowing through them. A fitting analogy would be the air conditioning found in an airplane: central cooling exists, but there are vents above each seat for passengers to control the airflow. Similarly, there is a system to regulate the blood flow of one organ alone, without creating a systemic change that would affect the entire body.

The arteries that supply the heart have a metabolic control mechanism. A metabolite called adenosine causes vasodilation in these vessels. Organs like the liver, gallbladder, pancreas and the intestines have their blood supply controlled by various hormones produced by the gut, kinins and bile acids released by the gallbladder. The kidneys produce urine by filtration of fluid and waste products from the blood. They can control the pressure by which the blood is filtered through the filtering body, called the glomerulus. The glomerulus is supplied by an afferent and an efferent arteriole. The two arterioles change in size to increase or decrease the blood pressure in the glomerulus.

Most organs in the body tend to vasodilate to increase the blood flow through them when oxygen concertation is low. The only organs that decrease their blood supply if the oxygen concentration is low, are the lungs. This is because the function of the lungs is to oxygenate the blood, and if a part of the lungs is damaged, say by pneumonia, then that part won't be able to oxygenate blood efficiently. Consequently, the vessels in the damaged part of the lung, or the part where oxygen concentration is low, constrict to decrease the blood supply to that area and to divert the flow of blood to the better-functioning areas of the lungs. This becomes problematic if the entire lung is damaged. If this is the case, the resistance of the vessels throughout the lung would increase, leading to pulmonary hypertension.

Cerebral blood flow, also called perfusion, denotes the volume of blood that passes through the brain capillaries to deliver oxygen and glucose to the brain cells, or the neurons. Despite its relatively small size, the brain uses about a quarter of the body's energy supply. Unlike other body organs that can metabolize other substances for energy, brain cells rely exclusively on glucose. This blood flow also removes wastes. Factors like carbon dioxide, oxygen and hydrogen ion concentrations influence blood flow changes within the brain. On an average, cerebral blood flow is 50 ml per 100 gm of brain tissue per minute, with blood flow in the grey matter being about four times that in the white matter. The brain requires approximately 500 ml of oxygen and 75–100 mg of glucose each minute, a total of around 125 gm of glucose each day. Cerebral blood flow is essentially stable across a wide range of systemic blood pressures due to arterial vasodilation and vasoconstriction. However, beyond a certain threshold, this blood flow depends on systemic blood pressure. For instance, if an individual has massive blood loss following a trauma or a problem with the heart, the brain will suffer damage due to the decreased blood supply.

Blood flow within the brain changes depending upon the activity of the neurons in a particular region. If an individual is speaking, the blood flow to the area of the brain that controls speech will increase.

The notion that blood flow is intimately related to brain function is surprisingly old. In 1878, Angelo Mosso, a prominent Italian physiologist, observed an increase in brain pulsations from the prefrontal cortex during an arithmetic task performed by a subject with a bony skull defect. In 1890, Charles Smart Roy and Charles Scott Sherrington first demonstrated the ability of the brain to increase local blood flow in response to the activity of the neurons in that region.

Despite this promising beginning, interest in the relationship between brain function and blood flow almost ceased during the first quarter of the twentieth century. This was due to the lack of sophisticated tools and the influence of Sir Leonard Hill, an eminent British physiologist who opposed the relationship between blood flow and brain function. In his 1896 book *The Physiology and Pathology of the Cerebral Circulation: An Experimental Research*, Hill rejected Roy and Sherrington's claims as inaccurate, considering his own experiments to be more precise.

There was no serious challenge to Leonard Hill's views until a remarkable clinical study of a patient, Walter K., was reported by John Fulton in a 1928 issue of the journal *Brain*. Walter K. had a vascular malformation over his visual cortex (the region of the brain that is located at the back and is associated with vision). He remarked to his physicians that a noise—a bruit—he perceived to originate in the back of his head increased when he was using his eyes. He said that he had often noticed this phenomenon during the preceding several years but had 'never thought much of it'. Fulton noticed that when the patient began to use his eyes after a period of prolonged rest in a dark room, there was a prompt and noticeable increase in the intensity of his bruit. The activity of his other sense organs had no effect upon the bruit. Fulton later became well-known for localizing cerebral function in primates. With Fulton's work and reputation, the theory correlating blood flow and brain function re-emerged. We now know that there is a designated area in the brain for a specific function. Different regions in the brain control different functions, like the visual cortex is for vision, the auditory cortex is for hearing and so forth. Modern techniques like positron emission tomography (PET) and functional MRI are based on this very concept of local changes in blood flow in the brain in response to regional activity. For instance, PET and MRI scans reveal that when a person raises their right hand, there is an increase in metabolism and blood flow in the left motor cortex (the region that controls the movement of the right hand) of the brain.

The presentation of stroke is the reverse. A particular vessel gets blocked, the area of the brain supplied by that vessel stops functioning and the patient presents with a loss of function pertaining to that brain region. For instance, if the blood vessel that supplies blood to the area that controls speech is blocked, the person will present with an inability to speak. Neurologists are trained to look at clinical signs that a patient presents with, then apply their knowledge of the brain's anatomy to localize the area of the brain that might be affected and identify the blood vessel supplying that area. As we know, most of the strokes are ischemic, caused by clots blocking the blood vessels. Using imaging techniques, the blocked vessels can be visualized and treated with drugs or interventional techniques which we will talk about in the subsequent chapters.

Now, it is worthwhile to know what forms these clots in the body that cause strokes. That knowledge is a gift of experiments conducted by another great personality as we shall see in the following chapter.

3

Virchow's Triad

For if medicine is really to accomplish its great task, it must intervene in political and social life. It must point out the hindrances that impede the normal social functioning of vital processes and effect their removal.

—Rudolf Virchow

I FIRST READ about Virchow's triad in the *Robbins Textbook of Basic Pathology*. We had four subjects during our second year of medical school: pharmacology (from *pharmakos*, meaning 'medicine' or 'drugs'), the study of various drugs; microbiology (from *mikros*, meaning 'small' and *bios*, meaning 'life'), the study of disease-causing organisms; pathology (from *pathologia*, meaning 'study of disease'), the study of the causes and effects of disease or injury; and forensic medicine (from *forēnsis*, meaning 'before the forum'), the application of medical and paramedical scientific knowledge to certain branches of both civil and criminal law.

The history of pathology can be traced back to the earliest application of scientific method to medicine. This development occurred in the Middle East during the Islamic Golden Age and in Western Europe during the Italian Renaissance. Hippocrates pioneered the study of anatomy and pathology of the human spine. Galen developed an interest in anatomy through his studies of Herophilus and Erasistratus. Although the concept of studying disease through the methodical dissection and examination of diseased bodies, organs and tissues may seem obvious today, there are few, if any, recorded examples of true autopsies performed prior to the second millennium. Though the pathology of contagion was understood by Muslim physicians since the time of Avicenna (980–1037 CE), who described it in *The Canon of Medicine* (c. 1020 CE), the first physician known to have done post-mortem dissections was the Arabian physician Avenzoar (1090–1162 CE), who proved that scabies, the skin disease, was caused by a parasite. This was followed by Ibn al-Nafis (1213–88 CE), who used dissection to discover pulmonary circulation in 1242 CE. In the fifteenth century, anatomic dissection was repeatedly used by the Italian physician Antonio Benivieni (1443–1502 CE) to determine the cause of death.

The most famous early gross pathologist was Giovanni Morgagni, who was born on 25 February 1682 in the small northern Italian town of Forlì. When he was sixteen, Morgagni went to the nearby city of Bologna to study medicine and philosophy. There, he came under the influence of the renowned anatomist Antonio Valsalva, who had been a pupil and disciple of Marcello Malpighi, a physician and biologist known for his study of microscopic anatomy. During his studies, Morgagni performed post-mortem examinations and kept notes on his cases. More than a year of graduate study followed, after which Morgagni returned to his hometown, Forlì, to become a practising physician. The years he spent practicing medicine in the small town were very productive and an important influence on his later career. He missed the academic environment that he had trained in, so in 1711, when he was invited to Padua to become a junior professor of theoretical medicine, he readily accepted. After four years of teaching and dissection, he earned the title of professor of anatomy at the University of Padua.

Morgagni assiduously collected cases that provided detailed histories of illnesses before death, along with autopsy examinations. His magnum opus, *De Sedibus et Causis Morborum per Anatomen Indagatis* (*The Seats and Causes of Diseases Investigated by Anatomy*), published in 1761, described the findings of over 600 partial and complete autopsies, organized anatomically and methodically correlated with the symptoms exhibited by patients prior to their death. Although the study of normal anatomy had been progressing steadily by this time (Andreas Vesalius's *De Humani Corporis Fabrica* was published in 1543), *De Sedibus* was one of the first treatises specifically devoted to the correlation of diseased anatomy with clinical illness. This wide gap between the first anatomical and pathological treatises was due to the nature of their subjects. Anatomy was the study of healthy body parts, which were easily accessible for observations. On the other hand, some rare pathological cases occurred only once during a physician's entire career. An anatomy treatise could be completed by the dissection of a small number of bodies, but to document various pathological lesions at different sites, a large number of bodies had to be dissected. Vesalius produced his anatomy treatise at the age of twenty-eight, whereas Morgagni was nearly eighty when he published *De Sedibus*, for which he relied on material assembled during his entire professional career and on reports collected by his teacher Valsalva. The extent of gross pathology research in the 1800s is epitomized by the work of the Austrian pathologist Carl Rokitansky (1804–78), who is said to have performed 20,000 autopsies and supervised an additional 60,000 in his lifetime.

It was Rudolf Ludwig Carl Virchow who dominated the field of medicine in the nineteenth century. Born on 13 October 1821 in Schievelbein, Eastern Pomerania (now part of Poland), he was the only child of a working-class family. He was remarkably intelligent and linguistically gifted, learning German, Dutch, Latin, Greek, Italian, Hebrew, English, Arabic and French in his lifetime. Virchow initially wanted to pursue theology but chose medicine instead, believing that his voice was too weak for preaching. In 1839, he received a military scholarship to study medicine at Friedrich-Wilhelm University in Berlin. He worked under Johannes Peter Müller, an eminent neurophysiological researcher whose studies improved the understanding of the sensory mechanisms governing vision and hearing. Müller's *Handbuch der Physiologie* (*Handbook of Physiology*) was referred to as the physiologist's bible. Under Müller's guidance, Virchow crafted a thesis on the corneal manifestations of rheumatic disease. Upon receiving his degree, Virchow wrote to his parents that he had received it from 'the world's most famous physiologist'. He then decided to intern at Berlin's Charité University Hospital, where he was mentored by Robert Froriep in microscopy. Virchow held the belief that medical progress was contingent upon making clinical observations, animal experimentation and studying pathological anatomy at the microscopic level.

In 1845, Virchow made a groundbreaking contribution by writing his first case report on 'leukemia', a term he coined for the presence of cancerous white cells in the blood. When several journal editors refused to publish two of his papers, Virchow, along with his colleague Benno Ernst Heinrich Reinhardt, founded a new journal in 1846: *Archiv für Pathologische Anatomie und Physiologie und für Klinische Medizin* (*Archives of Pathological Anatomy and Physiology and of Clinical Medicine*). The journal published research of the highest quality, with manuscripts with outdated, untested or speculative and dogmatic ideas being rejected. The journal was later renamed *Virchows Archiv* and is still published by the European Society of Pathology.

In 1848, Virchow was tasked with studying the typhus epidemic in Upper Silesia (today located mostly in Poland). Rather than just recommending better hygiene or sanitation, he suggested political freedom and social and educational reforms for the people. His political ideas infuriated the government, and he was forced to move from Berlin to Würzburg, where he spent the next seven years. However, his exile turned out to be rather productive, as during this period he deeply studied cells and contributed to the cell theory. He popularized the epigram *Omnis cellula e cellula*—all cells arise from pre-existing cells. He also studied venous thrombosis (the formation of blood clots in the veins). In 1856, Virchow returned to Charité University Hospital in Berlin as the director of the newly established pathological institute.

Virchow's work on thrombosis began when he was challenged by his professor Robert Froriep to counter the claim made by Cruveilhier that inflammation caused coagulation (the process of blood clotting). Virchow, who was sceptical of this idea, focused his experiments on the development of pulmonary thrombosis (blood clots found in the vessels of the lungs). A post-mortem examination led him to an astounding observation: the clots that he saw in the lungs had not originated in the lungs themselves but were parts of larger thrombi in the other distant vessels, such as the leg. The concave surface of the clot found in the lung fitted the larger clot in the leg perfectly: 'like a cap'. It seemed like the clot in the leg had broken into smaller parts that had travelled through the heart to the lungs.

To prove his hypothesis that clots travelled in the body through blood, Virchow proceeded to undertake experiments on dogs. He injected substances like cadaveric thrombi, coagulated blood and berries in the jugular veins of dogs to represent thrombi travelling from the legs. Many of his experimental dogs developed respiratory distress (i.e. difficulty in breathing) following the procedure, thus proving that blood could transport foreign substances to the lungs. Virchow termed this phenomenon 'embolism' and the detached clots 'emboli'. Inflammation, he believed, was a secondary process due to the chemical changes in the thrombus. Virchow also observed that clots were formed around an introduced foreign body, which he explained to be the consequence of irritation of the vessel wall, increased tendency of the blood to clot or obstruction to the flow of blood. These concepts formed the basis of 'Virchow's triad', which consists of three factors influencing thrombus formation:

1. Endothelial injury (injury to the vessel wall)
2. Blood hypercoagulability (increased tendency of the blood itself to clot)
3. Stasis or turbulence of blood flow

Along with pulmonary embolism, Virchow also investigated cerebral embolism (clots in the brain), which he considered to be the most common cause of 'ischemic' (his term) apoplexy. He thus reclassified apoplexy as 'sanguinea' (with intracerebral haemorrhage) and 'ischaemica' (due to occlusions, as with emboli). The most common sites of cerebral embolism were found to be the middle and anterior cerebral arteries, the carotid arteries and the vertebral arteries.

Virchow's work on thrombosis was superseded by his student Julius Cohnheim, who introduced emboli into the tongues of frogs by injecting wax globules in their arteries.

In his three-volume treatise on blood vessels, Virchow described the different abnormalities that can arise in the arteries and veins of the brain. His writings covered telangiectatic venous malformations, arterial malformations, arteriovenous malformations and cystic angiomas. Vascular malformations, as we know today, can cause haemorrhagic stroke.

Rudolf Virchow's legacy has led to him being known as 'the father of modern pathology'. He was not only a brilliant pathologist but also a physician, anthropologist and a politician. His contributions to medicine include the identification of Virchow's node, Virchow–Robin spaces, the phagocytic nature of neuroglia cells in encephalomalacia and tumours of the spinal cord. He also discovered the substance amyloid. Beyond pathology, Virchow contributed to parasitology, forensic medicine and anthropology.

Virchow continued to influence medicine internationally till his death in 1902. Even at eighty-one, his vigour remained, as evidenced when he jumped from a running streetcar. Unfortunately, this daring act resulted in a hip fracture that never fully healed, and his health began to deteriorate rapidly. He died soon after of heart failure.

4

The Heart and Brain Connection

Follow your heart but take your brain with you.

—Alfred Adler

HYPERTENSION AND STROKE

IN THE 1840S, while working in Vienna, the pathologist Carl Rokitansky introduced a novel concept: the link between heart disease and haemorrhagic apoplexy. Through autopsies, Rokitansky observed that individuals with bleeding in the brain were also found to have hypertrophy of the left ventricle of the heart. He therefore suggested that haemorrhage might arise from an increased 'impulse', what we recognize today as high blood pressure.

The heart has four chambers: the right atrium, right ventricle, left atrium and left ventricle. The right side of the heart receives deoxygenated blood from the body and pumps it to the lungs. Once oxygenated in the lungs, the blood moves into the left atrium, subsequently filling the left ventricle, which pumps it to the rest of the body. As hypertension develops, the diameters of the peripheral arteries become narrow and stiff. In order to pump blood through these resistant vessels, the left ventricle hypertrophies—it increases in bulk due to the thickening of the muscle fibres. This mirrors how muscles bulk up after exercising in the gym. Left ventricular hypertrophy is a very common finding in individuals with untreated hypertension and can also be traced on the electrocardiogram (ECG).

In 1868, Jean-Martin Charcot and his student Charles-Joseph Bouchard investigated the cause of spontaneous intracranial haemorrhage. They analysed the brain autopsies of eighty-four patients affected by haemorrhagic stroke. By macerating samples from fresh intracranial haemorrhage cavities in running water and washing away unclotted blood and parenchymal tissue, they were able to examine the vessels that caused the bleed under their microscope. They found miniscule 'milliary' (resembling millet seeds) aneurysms (*aneurysma*, meaning 'dilation') on the small perforating arteries supplying areas of the brain such as the basal ganglia, pons, cerebellum and cerebral white matter. These aneurysms were much smaller than the saccular aneurysms associated with subarachnoid haemorrhage (which we will explore in Chapter 9).

Charcot–Bouchard aneurysms, as they are called today, develop in the brain's very small arteries (less than 300 micron in diameter). They are a result of chronic hypertension, and are very small, balloon-like dilatations of the blood vessels that eventually expand and can rupture, causing haemorrhagic stroke.

Today, the majority of strokes are ischemic, with haemorrhagic strokes accounting for only 15–20 per cent of total strokes. Historically, this was not the case. When hypertension was not taken seriously and lacked effective treatments, haemorrhagic strokes were more common, so much so that apoplexy was almost synonymous with intracranial haemorrhage.

Hypertension as a distinct medical condition came into being in 1896 with the invention of the cuff-based sphygmomanometer by Scipione Riva-Rocci. This allowed blood pressure to be measured in the clinic. The technique was further improved by Nikolai Korotkoff, who described the characteristic sounds (now called Korotkoff sounds) that are heard when the artery is auscultated with a stethoscope while the sphygmomanometer cuff is deflated.

The historical treatment of hypertension, or 'hard pulse disease', was aimed at reducing blood volume through bloodletting or the application of leeches.

Many other non-pharmacological treatments were used in the late nineteenth and early to mid-twentieth centuries. These included strict salt restriction, injections of pyrogens such as typhoid bacilli, and various surgical methods such as sympathectomy and adrenalectomy. Sodium thiocyanate was the first chemical to be used for hypertension in the 1900s, but its use was limited due to high levels of toxicity. At the time, physicians did not recognize the importance of aggressive hypertension treatment.

It wasn't until President Franklin Roosevelt's death that the consequences of untreated hypertension gained public attention. Roosevelt was documented to have had hypertension since the age of fifty-four but did not receive treatment for another four years. He was later prescribed phenobarbital and massage therapy for a blood pressure of 188/105 mm Hg, in 1941. In February 1945, during the Yalta Conference, Roosevelt's health declined, with his blood pressure shooting up to 260/150 mm Hg. He exhibited signs of heart failure, had shortness of breath and lethargy. On the morning of 12 April 1945, Roosevelt complained of a severe headache while sitting for a portrait session. His blood pressure was recorded to be a staggering 300/190 mm Hg. He lost consciousness shortly after and died, succumbing to a haemorrhagic stroke, a result of his hypertension.

Roosevelt's death highlights a crucial issue: prior to World War II, there were few effective antihypertensive drugs and the available agents were poorly tolerated. The other agents used after the war were hexamethonium, hydralazine and reserpine. A breakthrough came with the discovery of the diuretic chlorothiazide, which was not only better tolerated but also prolonged the life of hypertensive patients. This was followed by the development of beta blockers by the British physician James Black in the early 1960s. The next class of drugs for hypertension were the calcium channel blockers, with verapamil being the pioneer drug of this class. As our understanding of the renin-angiotensin system in the regulation of blood pressure grew, many angiotensin-converting enzyme inhibitors were developed. More recently, angiotensin receptor blocking agents have been introduced as antihypertensive agents.

The early diagnosis and management of hypertension has significantly reduced the incidence of haemorrhagic strokes. When a patient presents with a haemorrhagic stroke, the initial management is aimed at reducing the patient's blood pressure with medication.

THE HEART AND ISCHEMIC STROKE

When it comes to ischemic strokes, a major source of the blood clots that block the arteries in the brain is the heart. Approximately 20 per cent of ischemic strokes are due to emboli from the heart, mainly from its left side. This is because blood from the left side of the heart goes to systemic circulation, whereas blood from the right side is pumped to the lungs.

Various conditions can cause clot formation in the chambers of the left heart, which are then pumped to the brain. The mechanism of clot formation aligns with Virchow's triad: hypercoagulability, stasis and endothelial injury.

In conditions such as atrial fibrillation, the heart's atria beat arrhythmically and at a rapid rate. This causes the blood flow in the heart to become turbulent, which results in endothelial dysfunction. It also forms counter currents with local pockets of stasis, this stasis leads to clot formation.

Additionally, conditions such as abnormal arterial dilatations can cause local stasis, leading to clot formation. Acute myocardial infarction (a heart attack) can also cause a remodelling of the ventricular wall and lead to abnormal dilatations that result in stasis and cardiac mural thrombi, which can then embolise and go to the brain. In other words, a heart attack can lead to a brain attack!

When the mitral valve, which connects the upper atrium of the heart to the lower ventricle, becomes stenosed, or narrow, it restricts blood flow. The atrium gets dilated due to the decreased blood flow rate to the ventricle, and this dilation can also cause stasis. Sometimes both abnormal dilation and irregular heart rhythms exist, drastically increasing the rate of clot formation in the heart. Consequently, individuals with these conditions might suffer multiple small strokes in various regions of the brain. Thus, in order to prevent both haemorrhagic and ischemic stroke, it is vital to maintain blood pressure and heart rhythm. Clot formation can be prevented using blood thinners, which are of two types: anticoagulants and antiplatelet drugs (discussed in Chapter 6).

The evaluation of the heart and its function is important in stroke patients as the heart is a frequent source of clots. The most commonly used tests to evaluate heart function are the electrocardiogram and the echocardiogram.

ELECTROCARDIOGRAM

In 1786, Luigi Galvani, an Italian physician at the University of Bologna, was the first to notice that electrical activity could be recorded in skeletal muscles, having demonstrated this phenomenon in a dissected frog's muscles. This observation would later inspire the naming of the 'galvanometer', an instrument used to measure and record electricity. In 1842, Carlo Matteucci, a professor of physics at the University of Pisa, used a frog as a model to demonstrate that electrical activity accompanies each heartbeat. Rudolf Albert von Kölliker and Heinrich Müller were the first to discover, in 1856, that the heart generated electricity. The first successful recording of electrical rhythm in the human heart seems to have been made by Alexander Muirhead between 1869 and 1870, using a siphon recorder at St. Bartholomew's Hospital, London. Remarkably, this equipment was originally devised to record signals passing through the first transatlantic cable, which had been laid in 1866.

In 1887, the British physiologist Augustus Desiré Waller postulated that there might be a way to record the electrical activity or voltage fluctuations of the human heart from the body's surface. In his experiments on both animals and humans, Waller found that the electrical currents generated by the heart could be recorded with a mercury capillary electrometer when the electrodes were placed on the chest or the limbs. This device was created in 1873 by the French physicist Gabriel Lippmann, who went on to receive the Nobel Prize in 1908 for his work on colour photography. The capillary electrometer utilizes a glass tube containing mercury. One end of the tube was drawn into a fine capillary and immersed vertically in diluted sulfuric acid. Measurement hinged on the displacement of the mercury meniscus; the mercury would expand or contract according to the potential difference between the mercury and the sulphuric acid, which were connected to electrodes on two separate points on the body. Waller indicated that the instrument reacted to as little as 1/40,000 of a volt.

Waller's pioneering demonstration of the human ECG (called the electrogram at the time) from an intact human heart took place at St. Mary's Hospital, London, in May 1887. He used surface electrodes strapped to the front and back of the chest. This early equipment showed only two distorted deflections: ventricular depolarization and repolarization. The P wave was not discernible at the time. Waller also used a number of other recording sites, including saline jars for limb immersion and, in one instance, placing an electrode on the left arm and a silver spoon in the mouth of the research subject. Waller frequently demonstrated the electrogram using his dog, Jimmy, who would stand with his paws in glass jars of saline. Surprisingly, Waller did not consider the idea of using his invention for clinical practice. He said in 1911, 'I do not imagine that electrocardiography is likely to find any very extensive use in the hospital ... It can at most be of rare and occasional use to afford a ... record of some rare anomaly of cardiac action.'

Willem Einthoven was born in 1860 in Java, Dutch East Indies (now Indonesia) and studied medicine at the University of Utrecht in the Netherlands. In 1887, he attended the International Congress of Physiology in London, where he saw Waller demonstrate the use of the capillary electrometer to record an electrograph of the heart. Inspired, Einthoven began to explore the use of the capillary electrometer to record minute electrical currents. By 1895, he had identified recognizable waves, which he labelled P, Q, R, S and T. The limitations of the capillary electrometer led Einthoven to devise a string galvanometer to record cardiac electrical activity. With his new technique, he standardized the tracings and formulated the concept of 'Einthoven's triangle', used in obtaining standard ECGs. In 1900, he concluded that the bioelectric signal of a diseased heart might differ from that of a healthy one. He described various abnormal findings on the electrocardiogram, such as bigeminy, complete heart block, P mitrale, right and left ventricular hypertrophy, atrial fibrillation and flutter, and the U wave. These specific abnormal findings on electrocardiograms help cardiologists in diagnosing various heart diseases.

Within ten years of Einthoven's clinical studies with the string galvanometer, the potential of electrocardiography was realized. Many arrhythmias were recognized and the association of T-wave inversion with angina and arteriosclerosis were identified in 1910. Einthoven is regarded as 'the father of electrocardiography' and was honoured with the Nobel Prize in Physiology or Medicine in 1924. Waller, having died in 1922, was ineligible for joint recognition.

ECHOCARDIOGRAPHY

The idea of echo reflection goes back to the end of the eighteenth century, when Lazzaro Spallanzani demonstrated that bats navigated using reflected echoes of inaudible sounds. In 1880, Pierre and Marie Curie discovered piezoelectricity, opening up the possibility of creating ultrasonic waves. The use of ultrasound for medical diagnostic purposes started in 1940. H. Gohr and T.H. Wedekin were the first to suggest the use of reflected ultrasound for the detection of tumours, abscesses and exudates. In 1946, French physiotherapist André Denier suggested the use of ultrasound to visualize structures located inside the human body. Interestingly, in 1947, the first image derived from the use of ultrasounds, by two Austrian brothers, the neurologist Karl Theodore Dussik and the physicist Friedrich Dussik, was of the brain's ventricles.

Inge Edler, the director of the cardiology department at Sweden's Lund University, was responsible for the preoperative evaluation of valvular heart disease. He sought to use ultrasound to diagnose the degree of mitral regurgitation (a condition in which the mitral valve, the valve between the left atrium and the left ventricle, doesn't close tightly, which allows blood to flow backwards into the heart) before performing heart surgery on patients with combined mitral valve disease. Upon discussing the challenge with a cardiac nurse, she suggested he speak to her husband, the physicist Jan Cederlund.

Cederlund put Edler in touch with his colleague and friend Carl Hellmuth Hertz, who had just completed reading an early version of the famous ultrasound book *Der Ultraschall*, to be included in his PhD studies. Even as a young boy, Hertz had been involved with ultrasound, helping his father, the Nobel Prize laureate in Physics in 1925, Professor Gustav Hertz, with the experimental work concerning Langevin radiation pressure. Because of this interest in ultrasound, Hertz was well acquainted with the Sperry Ultrasonic Reflectoscope developed by Floyd Firestone in the USA for non-destructive material testing. Thus, upon meeting with Edler and hearing about the cardiac question at issue, it occurred to him that this newly developed tool might be useful for measuring the expansion of the left atrium. Anticipating a 50 per cent chance of success, they began practical experiments without any prior knowledge of ultrasound's potential as a medical diagnostic tool.

Hertz knew that the first Ultrasonic Reflectoscope had been delivered to a company in Malmo responsible for non-destructive material testing at major shipyards. He travelled there to inspect this instrument, and when applying the transducer to the precordium (the portion of the body over the heart), he observed pulsatile echo signals. Encouraged by this positive result, the manager of the company lent the Reflectoscope to Lund University for a weekend in May 1953. In the laboratory of the Department of Medicine at the University Hospital in Lund, Hertz and Edler investigated several patients. The results were encouraging.

Edler and Hertz first reported the continuous recording of heart wall movements in 1954 and, by 1956, described the use of the ultrasonic cardiogram for diagnosing mitral valve disease.

To know exactly what cardiac structures he was studying with the ultrasound examination, Edler started by studying patients who were dying. He initially marked the location and direction of the ultrasonic beam, and after the patient's passing, he would perform an autopsy to correlate his examination findings with the actual structures. Edler identified several structures on the echocardiogram and produced a film about his findings, which was screened at the European Congress of Cardiology in 1960.

In 1977, Edler and Hertz were the joint recipients of the Lasker Award, considered the American counterpart to the Nobel Prize in Medicine. Today, they are cited as the fathers of echocardiography.

THE FRAMINGHAM HEART STUDY

During the first half of the twentieth century, there was a steady increase in deaths attributed to heart disease. However, the causes of coronary heart disease were speculative. Investigations comprised descriptive case reports and case-control comparisons of small studies.

This led to the Framingham Heart Study, an ongoing, long-term cardiovascular cohort study of residents of Framingham, Massachusetts. Launched in 1948 with 5,209 adult subjects, this study is now on its third generation of participants. These participants, and their children and grandchildren, voluntarily consented to undergo a detailed collation of their medical histories along with physical examinations and medical tests every three to five years, creating a wealth of data on physical and mental health, especially cardiovascular disease. A non-profit charity called Friends of Framingham Heart Study was founded to help defray study costs and spread awareness about heart issues. Fifty years' worth of data collected from the residents of Framingham has produced over 1,000 scientific papers. This vast body of research not only introduced the concepts of biological and environmental risk factors but also identified the major risk factors associated with heart disease, stroke and other diseases. It brought about a revolution in preventive medicine and forever changed how the medical community and the general population viewed the risk factors that led to certain diseases and how they could be prevented with lifestyle modifications or medications. Of note, the Framingham study was the first major cardiovascular study that included female participants. It marked a milestone in the history of cardiology and served as a model for many other longitudinal cohort studies.

The first report of this long-term study, 'Factors of risk in the development of coronary heart disease—six-year follow-up experience; the Framingham Study', was published in *Annals of Internal Medicine* in 1961. The study indicated that high blood pressure, smoking and high cholesterol levels were major factors in heart disease. It also emphasized the risk-reducing benefits of exercise and the negative impacts of obesity on heart health.

The study had been intended to last twenty years, and by 1968, it was debated whether the original study had served its purpose and should be terminated as scheduled. A committee gathered and considered that, after twenty years of research, the Framingham study should come to an end, since their hypothesis had been tested and extensive information concerning heart disease had been gathered. Despite this conclusion, Congress failed to accept the recommendation, instead voting to continue the study. In the decades that followed, the study continued to uncover profound observations. During the 1970s, it showed that elevated blood pressure increased the risk of stroke. It also highlighted that postmenopausal women had an increased risk of heart disease as compared to women who were premenopausal, and underscored the influence of psychosocial factors on heart disease risk.

In the 1980s, it was proved that HDL (good) cholesterol reduced the risk of heart disease. It also disproved the rumour that filtered cigarettes lower the risk of heart disease as opposed to non-filters.

The study delved even deeper in the 1990s, identifying that having an enlarged left ventricle of the heart increased the risk of stroke (an observation made by Rokitansky in the 1840s) and that elevated blood pressure could result in heart failure. Furthermore, this decade saw the introduction of the Framingham Risk Score, a tool that correctly predicted the ten-year risk for future coronary heart disease events in an individual.

In the 2000s, several other associations between risk factors and heart disease were recognized. The SHARe project was announced, a genome-wide association study with the Framingham Heart Study. The American Heart Association considers certain genomic findings of the Framingham Heart Study among the top research achievements in cardiology. Among these findings were genes linked to an increased risk of atrial fibrillation. The study also found that the risk of poor memory was increased in middle-aged men and women if their parents had suffered from dementia.

ATHEROSCLEROSIS

Arteriosclerosis (derived from the Greek *arteria*, meaning 'artery' and *sclerosis*, meaning 'hardening') is a general term describing any hardening and loss of elasticity of medium or large arteries. The more specific atherosclerosis (from *athera*, meaning 'gruel') is the hardening of an artery specifically due to an accumulation of atheromatous plaque—a build-up of fat, cholesterol, calcium and other substances found in the blood. This plaque leads to the narrowing of arteries, which limits the flow of oxygen-rich blood to various parts of the body. While atherosclerosis generally starts when a person is young, it typically worsens with age. Almost all people are affected by it to some degree by the age of sixty-five. Initially there are no symptoms, but if they occur, they generally do not begin before middle age. As atherosclerosis worsens, it can lead to heart attacks and strokes. It can also impact the peripheral arteries that supply blood to the legs, arms and pelvis, and can present as numbness and pain in the arms or legs. Another significant location for plaque formation is the renal arteries, which supply blood to the kidneys. Plaque occurrence and accumulation leads to decreased kidney blood flow and chronic kidney disease, which, like all other areas, are typically asymptomatic till their late stages. Today, atherosclerosis is the number one cause of death and disability in advanced economies.

In 1908, A.I. Ignatowski, in St. Petersburg, Russia, observed a possible relation between cholesterol-rich foods and experimental atherosclerosis. Two years later, Adolf Windaus found that atheromatous lesions contained six times as much free cholesterol as a normal arterial wall and twenty times more esterified cholesterol. Building on this, Nikolai Anichkov fed rabbits a cholesterol-rich diet (rabbits are herbivores; they only eat grass, fruits and vegetables and never cholesterol-rich foods) to induce atherosclerosis, and demonstrated that it was cholesterol alone that caused these atherosclerotic changes in the rabbits' arteries. He found early lesions such as fatty streaks as well as advanced lesions. He standardized cholesterol feeding and discovered that the amount of cholesterol uptake was directly proportional to the degree of atherosclerotic severity.

In 1950, the American physician and scientist John Gofman and his associates distinguished between low-density lipoprotein (LDL) cholesterol and high-density lipoprotein (HDL) cholesterol using the ultracentrifuge technique. In addition, they found that 101 of 104 men who had experienced heart attacks had elevated LDL molecules, a finding they had also observed in their cholesterol-fed atherosclerotic rabbits. Gofman's group observed an inverse relationship between HDLs and the risk of coronary artery disease.

In general, HDL is considered 'good' cholesterol, as it transports cholesterol to the liver for removal, while LDL is considered 'bad', as it takes cholesterol directly to the arteries.

In 1952, Laurence Kinsell and his colleagues found that consuming plant-based foods and avoiding animal fats decreased blood cholesterol levels. The most important study to identify blood cholesterol as a risk factor for coronary artery disease was the Framingham Study, which showed that the risk of developing clinically significant coronary disease was a continuous curvilinear function of blood cholesterol levels.

Many cholesterol-lowering agents were introduced into clinical use in the 1950s and '60s. These included nicotinic acid, cholestyramine, clofibrate and plant sterols. Recognizing the importance of dietary habits, the American Heart Association began encouraging people to follow a 'prudent diet' in 1961. A further understanding of cholesterol's metabolism was achieved by Konrad Bloch and Feodor Lynen, who received the Nobel Prize in Physiology or Medicine in 1964. During the 1970s, Michael Brown and Joseph Goldstein found the LDL receptor and the LDL pathway—a significant discovery that brought them the 1985 Nobel Prize in Physiology or Medicine. A major breakthrough in the management of increased blood cholesterol levels was the discovery of the group of drugs called 'statins'. The Japanese biochemist Akira Endo discovered the earliest statin, compactin, in 1976. Many vascular disease experts rate statins as the most important class of agents introduced into medicine during the last half century. Studies have shown that treatment with statins lowers blood LDL levels by 25–35 per cent and reduces the frequency of heart attacks by 25–30 per cent. The international Stroke Prevention by Aggressive Reduction in Cholesterol Levels (SPARCL) trial led by French neurologist Pierre Amarenco, underscored the effectiveness of statins in stroke prevention.

5

No-Man's Land

The two branches which they call carotids or soporales, the sleepy arteries, because they being obstructed, or any way stopped, we presently fall asleep.

—Ambroise Paré

THE COMMON CAROTID artery in the neck bifurcates into the internal carotid artery, which enters the skull, and the external carotid artery, which caters predominantly to the facial tissues. The term 'carotid' comes from the Greek *karos*, which means 'to stun, stupefy or fall into deep sleep'—a reflection of ancient observations that superficial compression of these arteries resulted in the loss of consciousness.

In med school, our professors often told us to auscultate the carotid arteries by placing the stethoscope on the patient's neck to detect any carotid bruit. A bruit, as mentioned earlier, is an abnormal sound generated by turbulent blood flow in an artery. This turbulence might arise due to an obstruction in the artery or a high rate of blood flow through an unobstructed artery. I never really understood its significance then, as my focus was always on the heart or the brain. Carotid artery disease occurs as a result of atherosclerosis (plaque deposition) in the carotids. Plaques are usually composed of cholesterol, calcium and cellular debris. Carotid artery disease can lead to a stroke, if the artery gets very narrow, leading to decreased blood flow, or via plaque rupture with its fragments blocking the smaller arteries of the brain. A blood clot can also form over the plaque, blocking the artery, and can cause an embolism elsewhere. With carotid artery disease affecting one side, the eye on the same side manifests symptoms. And since one side of the brain controls the opposite side of the body, symptoms would appear on the opposite side of the rest of the body. For example, right-sided carotid artery disease would cause transient blindness in the right eye and a paralysis of the body's left side.

The understanding of carotid artery disease as a cause of stroke was hit upon in the 1950s, a revelation largely attributed to the brilliance of Charles Miller Fisher, who was both a clinician and a neuropathologist.

Born in 1913 in Waterloo, Ontario, Canada, Fisher was one among nine siblings. Soon after graduating from the University of Toronto's Faculty of Medicine in 1938, he wed Doris, who went on to be his wife of sixty-eight years. In 1940, as war engulfed Europe, he volunteered for the Canadian Navy. However, heeding the United Kingdom's urgent call for more naval medical officers, he was seconded to the British Royal Navy. In 1941, his dedication was tested while he was the ship doctor on an armed merchant cruiser called the *Voltaire*. When a German vessel attacked and damaged the *Voltaire* in the South Atlantic, the ship tilted precariously, forcing the crew to abandon it. Lifeboats could not be launched because of the angle of the list, so the survivors had to jump or slide into the (fortunately) warm waters, being plucked out of the ocean by the enemy over six hours later. Fisher was forced to spend the next three and a half years as a physician in a German prisoner-of-war camp, where he taught himself German. He was repatriated in September 1944 as one of the supervising doctors involved in an exchange of wounded prisoners of war.

When he resumed his medical career in Canada, Fisher's intention was to focus on diabetes and metabolic diseases. However, as part of a medical refresher course, he had a rotation at the Montreal Neurological Institute–Hospital, where, during morning bedside rounds, he came to the attention of Wilder Penfield, MD, the institute's legendary director. Penfield quickly recognized Fisher's inquiring mind and became his mentor. He arranged for a residency position for Fisher at the institute and subsequently encouraged Fisher to pursue a neuropathology fellowship with Raymond D. Adams, MD, at Boston City Hospital. By the age of thirty-six, Fisher had made his way back to Montreal to assume the role of a neuropathologist at Montreal General Hospital.

Unfortunately, before the advent of tools like CT or MRI, many medical diagnoses would be made at the autopsy table and carotid artery occlusion as the cause of stroke was often missed. As explained by Fisher, 'Clinicians and physicians have heretofore failed to appreciate this condition, because the cervical portion of the carotid artery lies on a "no-man's land" between general pathology and neuropathology, its examination at autopsy being therefore neglected.' Thus, the brain and other organs were examined in detail, but nobody bothered looking in the neck.

While working at Queen Mary Veterans Hospital, Montreal, in 1950, Fisher encountered a sixty-eight-year-old male patient with left hemiplegia (paralysis of the left side of the body). Two months prior to the hemiplegia, he had experienced five or six episodes of transient blindness in the right eye. He remarked to Fisher, 'Isn't it funny that I went blind in the wrong eye? My paralysis is on the left side and it was my right eye that went blind.' One week later, Fisher had another patient with a similar stroke that was preceded by multiple episodes of blindness in one eye. These two cases led him to consider the possibility of a thrombotic process in the carotid arteries. Two or three months later, Fisher's first patient died while he was away one weekend. Upon returning on Monday, he found that no autopsy had been conducted as the resident on call had not considered it necessary. The family had actually asked if the autopsy needed to be done! Reluctantly, Fisher called the patient's wife to ask for permission to perform an autopsy. Thankfully, she agreed, allowing the procedure to take place at the funeral home. At eleven that night, Fisher and the funeral director did the autopsy and for the first time took out the carotids. On cutting the right carotid, he found it to be occluded. Thus, he substantiated his clinical diagnosis with pathological examination.

Fisher went on to emphasize the frequent occurrence of warnings before stroke, which he later dubbed transient ischemic attacks. 'Prodromal fleeting attacks of paralysis, numbness, tingling, speechlessness, unilateral blindness, or dizziness often preceded and warned of impending strokes in patients with carotid artery disease,' he noted.

To further his understanding, he began routinely examining the carotids, analysing around 1,100 pairs of carotids over the next three years. He established the correlation between prodromal symptoms, such as transient ischemic attacks of blindness, and strokes. He also suggested the use of anticoagulant therapy using heparin and coumarin derivatives to arrest transient ischemic attacks. Looking ahead, he speculated about the role of surgery in bypassing blocked portions of the artery: 'It is even conceivable that someday vascular surgery will find a way to bypass the occluded portion of the artery during the period of ominous fleeting symptoms. Anastomosis of the external carotid artery or one of its branches with the internal carotid artery above the area of narrowing should be feasible.'

In 1954, Raymond D. Adams was asked to develop a neuromedical service at Massachusetts General Hospital (MGH). He invited Fisher to return to Boston to join him. There began an intensive collaboration that ultimately impacted the construct and culture of neurology, including the recognition of stroke disease as primarily a neurologic, rather than an internal medicine problem. Fisher spent the next half century at MGH and Harvard University, where he created and led the first formal stroke service. Many of his stroke service trainees became global leaders in the stroke field, including my mentor, Dr Louis R. Caplan.

Dr Caplan often recounted a story told to him by Dr Fisher in the early 1960s. While having lunch with three cardiologists, Fisher shared with them an observation from his latest autopsies. He had found brain embolism in patients with atrial fibrillation but who had no valvular disease and suggested atrial fibrillation as a cause of stroke. The three experienced cardiologists ignored the suggestion and asserted that they had many atrial fibrillation patients and were aware of no strokes. In a twist of fate, all three of those very cardiologists eventually developed atrial fibrillation and brain embolism.

Fisher's contributions were not limited to the discovery of carotid stenosis but extended to the identification of carotid dissection as a cause of stroke; the demonstration that atrial fibrillation was a frequent stroke substrate and that initial strokes owing to atrial fibrillation were often catastrophic; the recognition of the clinical and pathologic features of thalamic and cerebellar haemorrhage; the identification of the syndromes of lacunar infarction; and the formulation of the Fisher score for aneurysmal subarachnoid haemorrhage.

Beyond the realm of strokes, Fisher's influence permeated general neurology. He is credited with identifying and describing various syndromes and phenomena, such as the Miller Fisher syndrome, normal pressure hydrocephalus, transient global amnesia, one-and-a-half syndrome, wrong-way eyes, pontine ptosis, oval pupils and rostral-caudal brain deterioration.

CAROTID LIGATION TO ENDARTERECTOMY

In 1552, French barber surgeon Ambroise Paré performed the first known carotid artery ligation to control bleeding in a wounded French soldier. Though the soldier's life was saved, he ended up developing aphasia and hemiplegia (the procedure stopped the bleeding but ligating the carotid artery compromised blood supply to that side of the brain causing the patient to develop one-sided paralysis and loss of speech). Hebenstreit of Germany, in 1793, recorded how he had accidently injured a carotid artery while excising a tumour. The bleeding was controlled by the ligation of the carotid and the patient lived for several more years. In 1798, John Abernethy reported to have ligated the common carotid artery to control bleeding in a man gorged by the horn of a cow. In 1803, David Fleming, a naval surgeon, performed successful ligation in a servant who had attempted suicide by cutting his own throat. Sir Astley Cooper's 1805 procedure marked a significant advance: he was the first to perform carotid artery ligation for the treatment of an aneurysm. An aneurysm is a weakening of the arterial wall, causing it to distend or bulge. Aneurysms can be seen as a swelling and can rupture, leading to massive bleeding.

As Cooper wrote:

> Mary Edwards, aged 44, was brought to my house by Mr Robert Pugh of Gracechurch Street, that I might examine a tumour in the neck which was obviously an aneurysm of the right carotid artery. While the swelling was examined at the hospital, great doubts were entertained if there were sufficient space between the clavicle and the tumour for the application of a ligature.

Charles Miller Fisher established the link between the occlusion of the internal carotid artery and the onset of stroke through his landmark papers published in 1951 and 1954. Attempts to restore cerebral circulation by surgically reconstructing the carotid arteries began soon after.

The first carotid artery reconstruction was performed by Raúl Carrea and his colleagues at the Institute of Biology and Experimental Medicine in Buenos Aires, Argentina, in 1951. Their patient was a fifty-one-year-old man with difficulty in speaking and right-sided hemiparesis. The patient underwent two angiographic studies and was operated two weeks after admission. The diseased portion of the internal carotid artery was cut out and the two ends were reconnected, which re-established blood flow. The surgery was successful, and the patient had normal findings on neurological examinations done thirty-nine months later.

Carotid endarterectomy is a procedure in which the plaque obstructing the artery is separated from the arterial wall and removed. The first carotid endarterectomy was performed by Michael DeBakey in 1953; however, he only reported this groundbreaking procedure in 1975, after following up with the patient for nineteen years. The patient, a fifty-two-year-old male bus driver, had been experiencing intermittent episodes of weakness in the right arm and leg, hesitancy and difficulty in speaking and difficulty in writing. The pulsations in the left (opposite side) carotid artery were extremely weak, while they were normal on the right side. A diagnosis of occlusion of the left internal carotid artery was made. On 7 August 1953, the patient was administered general anaesthesia and his left common, internal and external carotid arteries were exposed through an incision in the neck. An occluding clamp was placed below the artery to stop the blood flow through it during the procedure. A cut was made in the internal carotid artery and yellowish-brown plaque was removed. The flow was restored in the artery and heparin was injected to prevent clot formation during the procedure. The arterial wall was then sutured using silk sutures. Strong pulses were felt in the arteries and the wound in the neck was closed in layers. The patient was followed up for nineteen years until his death due to heart disease.

A similar procedure was performed by Denton Cooley in March 1956, on a seventy-one-year-old man who had complaints of a 'swishing' noise in his left ear for four months. A unique aspect of Cooley's approach was the immersion of the patient's head in crushed ice to prevent brain damage due to the temporary interruption of blood supply during the procedure. (Immersing the head in crushed ice decreased the temperature and slowed the brain's metabolism and hence its demand for oxygen while the blood supply was interrupted during the procedure).

Today, the treatment of carotid artery disease has diversified. Modern options include medical therapy, carotid endarterectomy and carotid artery stenting, where a stent is placed in the artery to prevent it from narrowing.

6

Blood Thinners

Look for something, find something else, and realize that what you've found is more suited to your needs than what you thought you were looking for.

—*Lawrence Block*

PREVENTING STROKES OFTEN hinges on reducing the body's tendency to form clots, and for this, various drugs can be administered. The two categories of drugs are: anticoagulants and antiplatelets. The aim is to prevent the formation of blood clots in the heart and the aorta, and in any regions of vascular narrowing and irregularity. Although these drugs are called 'blood thinners', they do not really change the thickness or viscosity of the blood; instead, they make the blood flowing in the vessels less likely to clot. These drugs play a delicate balance, though: while they are used to prevent ischemic strokes, they increase the risk of bleeding, since they reduce blood clotting. This means they can cause or worsen a haemorrhagic stroke. Consequently, their administration is nuanced, and doctors tailor them for individual patients. Some drugs require regular monitoring so that their levels remain optimal, neither too low to cause blood clotting nor too high to increase the risk of bleeding.

Some of the commonly used anticoagulant drugs are heparin, warfarin, rivaroxaban, dabigatran and apixaban. There are a total of twelve different molecules or blood-clotting factors that are involved in blood clotting. The same way a sticker has a protective strip of paper that is peeled off to reveal the adhesive, these twelve factors move in the blood in an 'inactive' state. Whenever there is a stimulus for blood to clot, such as tissue injury, the coagulation cascade is activated: different clotting factors are triggered and lead to clot formation by converting inactive 'fibrinogen' (the suffix *gen* means 'that which produces') into active fibrin, a protein that forms the basic meshwork of a clot. The anticoagulants prevent this production of fibrin by acting on various clotting factors (depending on the drug) in the blood and blocking the coagulation cascade (see figure 5).

Antiplatelet drugs, on the other hand, alter the function of blood platelets. When an artery becomes irregular and plaque forms, the altered inner lining of the blood vessels stimulates the platelets in the blood to stick to the surface of the plaque and to one another by using fibrin. This results in the creation of white clots, formed of platelets and fibrin, which can embolize vessels and cause transient ischemic attacks or strokes. Platelet activation can also stimulate the formation of a superimposed red clot made of red blood cells mixed with fibrin. Some of the commonly used antiplatelet drugs are aspirin, clopidogrel, dipyridamole, cilostazol and abciximab.

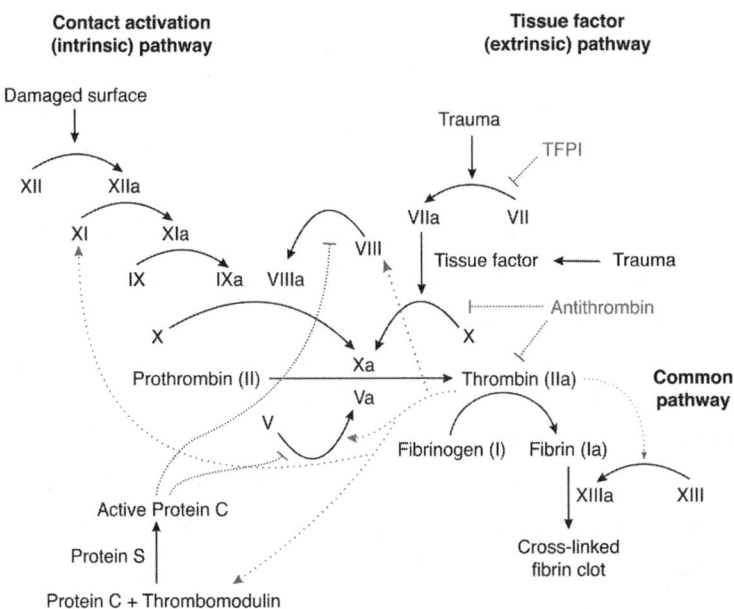

Figure 5 The coagulation cascade, showing how various factors are activated by two different pathways and lead to clot formation.

THE STORY OF HEPARIN

In 1880, a German researcher named Schmidt-Mulheim described how mammals could, in all probability, possess indigenous anticoagulants. Then, in 1905, Morawitz reviewed the research on peptone shock and concluded that a definitive characterization of the anticoagulant could not be arrived at on the basis of the analytic methods prevalent at that time. Further progress on this subject was made almost a decade later by Howell and McLean.

William Henry Howell was born in Baltimore, Maryland, in 1860 and was educated in local schools, where his interest in chemistry and medicine blossomed. While in his third year of high school, he accepted a paid position as an assistant to a natural sciences teacher, which gave him the opportunity to perform experiments. In 1879, he enrolled in Johns Hopkins University and fulfilled the requirements for a PhD in Biology in 1884. His dissertation, titled 'Experiments upon the Blood and Lymph of the Terrapin and the Origin of the Fibrin Formed in the Coagulation of Blood', examined the molecular components involved in the generation of a blood clot and isolated thrombin and fibrinogen. He observed that the addition of thrombin to fibrinogen generated a fibrin clot.

In 1889, Howell accepted an appointment at the University of Michigan as chairman of the Department of Physiology. He returned to Johns Hopkins University four years later to become the first professor of physiology. Beyond being an outstanding teacher, he was a devoted experimentalist. His contributions were recognized when he became a charter member of the American Physiological Society, founded by various well-known physiologists. Howell wrote a textbook on human physiology, *A Textbook of Physiology for Medical Students and Physicians,* which went through an impressive fourteen editions.

Born in San Francisco in 1890, Jay McLean faced significant adversities from childhood. He lost his father when he was just four years old. About a decade later, fifteen-year-old McLean and his family were ruined when the infamous 1906 San Francisco earthquake ravaged the city. Despite the chaos, McLean joined the University of California at Berkeley in 1909, and while there decided to pursue a career in academic surgery at Johns Hopkins Medical School. He wrote in his autobiography, 'I deliberately chose the fiercest student competition as Johns Hopkins' matriculants were meticulously chosen.'

In 1913, he commenced his final year at the University of California, which was concurrently his first year as a medical student, and graduated in 1914. During that pivotal first year studying medicine, McLean was introduced to physiology. The textbook they used was penned by none other than William Henry Howell. McLean was fascinated by the subject and its research possibilities, and applied for admission to Johns Hopkins for his second year, but his application was denied.

Nevertheless, he decided to move to Baltimore and met with the registrar and the dean, who were surprised to see him and inquired if he had not received the letter denying him admission. He candidly told them that his plan was to work for a year and then try again. Fortunately, the very next day, word was sent to him that there was an unexpected vacancy and that he was admitted to the school for his second year of medicine.

McLean's drive pushed him to approach Professor Howell. He expressed his desire to devote an entire year to physiological research. At the time, Howell was trying to determine the value of clot-promoting agents from different tissues. He had obtained a thromboplastic (clot-promoting) substance, which was a mixture of macerated brain tissue called 'cephalin' (from *cephal*, meaning 'head'). He assigned McLean the task of determining the portion of the crude extract that activated the clotting process and to prepare cephalin as pure as possible. Meanwhile, McLean also took an advanced course in German to better understand German chemistry literature, as he had found some German articles on phosphatides by Erlandsen and Baskoff in which they described the extracts of the heart and liver secured by a process similar to that used to obtain cephalin from the brain. The extract from the heart was called 'cuorin' and that from the liver was called 'hepraphosphatide' (from *hepar*, meaning 'liver').

Though the process of extraction was the same for the brain, heart and liver tissues, the end products differed. While the brain yielded pure cephalin, the heart and liver extracts contained something else mixed with cephalin. McLean saved batches of extracts for months and upon retesting them found that the extract from the liver (more than from the heart) possessed a strong anticoagulant action after its contained cephalin had lost its thromboplastic action.

Howell was not convinced of McLean's discovery of an anticoagulant. So, McLean got a beaker full of cat's blood and stirred all of a proven batch of hepraphosphatides into it. He placed the beaker on Howell's laboratory table and asked him to tell him when it clotted. To Howell's astonishment, it never did.

In 1916, McLean published his paper 'The Thromboplastic Action of Cephalin'. In it, he discussed the thromboplastic properties of cephalin and its preparation from the liver, heart and brain. He did not conduct any further research on anticoagulants as his research year had ended and redirected his focus on completing medical school.

Howell, however, carried on the research on the anticoagulant hepraphosphatide with Emmett Holt. In 1918, Howell and Holt named this substance 'heparin' and described a method for its extraction from dried dog liver.

But using dog liver was unsuitable for large-scale production, so the purification process was greatly improved in Toronto during the 1930s by Arthur F. Charles and David A. Scott. They shifted the tissue source from dog or cow liver to cow lung, which was cheaper and gave higher yields. Beef lung became the main source material for heparin production until the 1950s, when it was largely replaced by porcine mucosa. Charles H. Best, known for conducting experiments with Frederick Banting that led to the discovery of insulin, worked closely with Charles and Scott to improve the manufacturing process at Connaught Laboratories, Toronto. Although their method required sixty-six separate steps, it culminated in a commercially viable method that used ox lung as a source. By 1937, heparin was available for use on a small scale. Even today, heparin is largely animal derived, though a variety of strategies, like microbial production, mammalian cell production and chemoenzymatic modification, have been proposed to produce a bioengineered heparin.

Heparin's injection-based administration limits its long-term use in patients. It is most commonly used to prevent strokes in patients with atrial fibrillation. It is also used in patients who have had cardiogenic emboli and are at risk for recurrence. While the anticoagulant warfarin has the advantage of being given orally, it takes a few days for its therapeutic action to begin, so heparin is used as a form of 'bridge therapy'—the patient is started on heparin first and then slowly transitioned to warfarin.

The clinically used antidote of heparin is protamine sulphate. The ability of protamine to reverse the anticoagulant effect of heparin was reported by Chargaff and Olson in New York. Protamine (also known as salmine, as it was once obtained from salmon roe) prolonged the effect of insulin. Interestingly, researchers expected protamine to have a similar prolongation effect on heparin. Instead, it turned out to be a potent antagonist.

THE STORY OF WARFARIN

In the 1920s, ranchers in northern USA and in Canada reported a mysterious condition causing their cattle to bleed to death following minor procedures, such as dehorning or castration; some even bled spontaneously, following no procedure. There was no identifiable pathogen or nutritional deficiency causing the bleeding. This mystery drew the attention of a Canadian veterinary pathologist, Dr Frank Schofield.

After some investigation, Schofield found a common factor among the affected cattle: they had eaten mouldy silage from a sweet clover plant. Sweet clover was a popular source of fodder since it grew in nutrient-poor soil and was a great source of protein. However, in damp weather, the silage became infected with *Penicillium nigricans* and *Penicillium jensi* mould. Schofield fed healthy clover hay stalks to one rabbit and mouldy ones to another. The rabbit that had consumed the spoilt hay died. Thus, Schofield demonstrated the anticoagulant properties of spoilt sweet clover hay, and the haemorrhagic disease came to be known as sweet clover disease.

The disease was found to be reversible upon abstinence from toxic sweet clover hay and by the administration of fresh blood to the animal. Farmers were advised to stop feeding their cattle mouldy sweet clover hay, but the exact chemical agent responsible for causing the disease could not be isolated from sweet clover.

The biochemist Karl Paul Gerhard Link was first introduced to sweet clover disease in December 1932, by Ross A. Gortner, the head of the biochemistry department of the University of Minnesota. In January 1933, Link began his research on sweet clover in collaboration with R.A. Brink and W.K. Smith of the genetics department of the university. However, their initial focus was not on finding the haemorrhagic agent in sweet clover but on genetically modifying the plant. They wanted a strain that was suitable for Wisconsin's climate and had a low coumarin content, for coumarin was the substance in sweet clover that made the plant taste bitter. The change of the course of Link's research was rather dramatic.

In February 1933, on a Saturday afternoon, a farmer named Ed Carlson approached Link. He had brought with him a dead cow, a milk can full of unclotted blood and about 100 pounds of sweet clover as 'evidence'. Several of his cows and bulls had succumbed to incessant bleeding, and he was at the end of his rope. While Link simply recommended stopping the use of the spoilt clover as cattle feed and suggested blood transfusions as a last resort, Eugen Wilhelm Schoeffel, one of Link's students, overheard the conversation. He persuaded Link to study the disease. Link, along with his students Smith, Roberts and Campbell, began the pursuit of the agent in sweet clover that was causing bleeding. In 1939, they isolated the compound dicumarol, which was a derivative of the compound coumarin— the one that was responsible for the bitter taste of the plant. In the next four years, Link and his students synthesized over a hundred related compounds. These coumarin derivatives were given numbers based on their chemical structure.

In early September 1945, while on vacation, Link had a relapse of tuberculosis. He spent two months at Wisconsin General Hospital and then got transferred to Lakeview Sanatorium. While there, he saw that the building had a rodent problem and urgently needed rat poison. He contemplated the use of a coumarin derivate as a rat poison. The agent numbered forty-two was proposed for rodenticidal use in 1948. It was named warfarin—'warf' from the Wisconsin Alumni Research Foundation, which funded their research, and 'arin' from coumarin. Warfarin turned out to be an excellent rat poison. Its delayed action meant that bait refusal (where rats avoid bait associated with the sudden deaths of other rats in the colony) was not an issue.

Clinicians were initially not in favour of using warfarin as an anticoagulant in humans. This changed after an incident on 5 April 1951, when an army inductee attempted suicide by consuming warfarin designed for rodent control. He had followed the multiple-dosage instructions on the package and consumed 567 mg of warfarin in corn starch over a period of five days. He was admitted to the naval hospital as a case of full-blown 'sweet clover disease'. Apparently, he got 'too much time to think', so he walked into the hospital. He recovered following blood transfusions and vitamin K administrations. In 1955, President Dwight Eisenhower, while on holiday in Denver, suffered a heart attack. He was initially treated with heparin but was then eventually started on warfarin at a dose of 35 mg per week.

Warfarin works by inhibiting the action of vitamin K, which is necessary for the biological synthesis of blood-clotting factors II, VII, IX and X. The therapeutic dosing window for warfarin is the range at which it effectively prevents thromboembolism that will cause ischemic stroke without causing a high rate of bleeding. Warfarin metabolism varies widely among and within individual patients and is influenced by other drugs, diet and, in women, hormonal fluctuations, such as with menstruation, pregnancy or the use of oral contraceptive pills. Accordingly, the regular monitoring of warfarin activity is necessary for its safe use.

To monitor the coagulation tendency in patients taking warfarin-type anticoagulants, certain blood tests, called prothrombin time determinants, are employed. These tests measure a patient's coagulation speed against normal standards. Results are expressed in time, for example fifteen seconds, and then compared to local controls in that lab. For example, it could be twice or thrice the time taken by the control to clot. The result can also be given as a ratio by comparison with an international standard, the International Normalized Ratio (INR). For patients with atrial fibrillation, the advised warfarin dosage aims to maintain an INR of 2.0–3.0. Higher doses of warfarin are needed for the prevention of cardiac emboli arising from mechanical mitral valve replacements, with a recommended INR target of 2.5–3.5.

THE STORY OF ASPIRIN

Ancient medical practitioners believed in the 'doctrine of signatures', which stated that natural objects that resembled parts of the body could cure diseases affecting those parts. For instance, the eyebright plant was used to cure eye diseases because its flowers resembled blue eyes. It was believed that the herbs were given particular 'signatures' by God for humans to identify and use them. Though this doctrine did not have any scientific basis, it did lead to the discovery of one of the most widely used drugs in the modern world: aspirin.

Ancient Egyptian records, such as the Ebers Papyrus, document the use of willow leaves for the treatment of inflammatory rheumatic diseases and as a pain killer. Hippocrates administered willow leaf tea to women to assuage the pain of childbirth. The first scientific description of the beneficial effects of the bark of the willow tree was given by the natural philosopher Reverend Edward Stone in a letter to the president of the Royal Society in 1763. He recalled tasting the bark in 1757 and being surprised by its extreme bitterness, similar to Peruvian bark (the source of quinine, used to treat malaria). He saw the bark of the willow tree as a potential cure for ague (malarial fever), based on the doctrine of signatures. He gathered a pound of the bark, dried it in a bag placed in front of a baker's oven for three months and then pulverized it. Cautiously, he administered very small quantities of the powder to a patient every four hours and found the symptoms of malaria to abate. He gradually increased the dose and found that the 'ague was removed'. Over five years, he successfully treated around fifty patients with this approach.

In 1828, Johann Andreas Buchner succeeded in isolating the active ingredient in willow bark in the form of bitter-tasting yellow crystals. He named the compound salicin (which means 'willow' in Latin). Ten years later, an Italian chemist, Raffaele Piria, succeeded in splitting the glycoside salicin to produce salicylic acid. In 1859, Hermann Kolbe, a professor of chemistry at the University of Marburg, identified the chemical structure of salicylic acid and synthesized it artificially. This facilitated the industrial production of salicylic acid, and by 1874, a factory in Dresden was selling it at one-tenth the price of the material extracted naturally.

In 1876, Thomas John MacLagan's paper detailing the first clinical trial on the efficacy of salicin to treat the pain and inflammation caused by rheumatic fever was published by *The Lancet*. He started with self-administration of the drug and, convinced of no ill-effects, began administering it to patients and reported its success in the treatment of eight cases of rheumatism. In his article, he urged other practitioners to report their experiences with the drug. Six weeks later, his appeal was answered by Frederick Ensor, a South African surgeon, who shared his experience of a patient who had full-blown rheumatic disease. He had prescribed the patient the usual alkaline mixture, calomel and Dover's powder at bedtime. Two months later, the patient returned, cured, but with the news that Ensor's medication hadn't helped her at all. The ameliorant had been a decoction made by a shepherd from the willows growing on the banks of the local river!

In 1897, Heinrich Dreser was put in charge of testing the efficacy and safety of new drugs at the pharmaceutical company Bayer. During his tenure as the head of the company, Bayer launched two drugs: the world's most successful legal drug, aspirin, and the most successful illegal drug, heroin.

During Dreser's tenure, Arthur Eichengrün was the head of the group creating new drugs. While salicylic acid was widely used for the treatment of rheumatic fever, many patients became intolerant to it because it had an unpleasant taste and caused severe stomach irritation. Eichengrün instructed Felix Hoffman, a chemist at Bayer, to work on a more tolerable form of salicylic acid. Coincidently, Hoffman's father was taking salicylic acid for his rheumatism and had severe side effects. Hoffman succeeded in devising a process for the acetylation of the phenol group of salicylic acid to produce acetylsalicylic acid, or ASA, which would later be named aspirin.

When Eichengrün proposed commercializing ASA, Dreser rejected it, fearing that it would have an 'enfeebling' action on the heart. Dreser's decision potentially stemmed from his interest in another drug, heroin, for he saw in it the potential to replace morphine as a non-addictive painkiller for respiratory distress. Heroin, whose chemical name is diacetylmorphine, was synthesized by Hoffman two weeks after he synthesized ASA. Dreser knew that it was first discovered by the English chemist Charles Romley Alder Wright, but he claimed it to be a Bayer invention. He tested the drug on various animals, workers and even himself, and was elated with the results. The workers reported that the drug made them feel 'heroic', hence the name heroin. Due to its sedative nature, the drug became popular as a 'cough remedy' for tuberculosis and pneumonia, which were prevalent then. By 1899, Bayer was exporting heroin to twenty-three countries in the form of heroin pastilles, cough lozenges, tablets and elixirs. The success of the drug was, however, transient, as researchers began reporting cases of addiction.

The company then shifted its focus to ASA and began testing the drug. Dreser tested it on himself and laboratory rabbits, and published a paper highlighting its use for the treatment of rheumatism. He did not mention the contributions of Hoffman or Eichengrün. The compound was then marketed as Aspirin (the 'a' coming from acetyl and the 'spir' from *spirea ulmania*, the plant from which salicylic acid was first isolated). Since the company could not market the drug directly to the public, Bayer circulated small packets of the drug to more than 30,000 doctors and encouraged them to prescribe it. By 1940, the powdered form of the drug was replaced by tablets stamped with Bayer's logo. This was done to establish a connection between Bayer and Aspirin and to distinguish it from competitors.

Dreser himself was rumoured to be addicted to heroin. He eventually succumbed to a stroke. Perhaps this stroke could have been prevented if he had been addicted to aspirin instead. The idea that aspirin could prevent heart attacks first occurred to Lawrence L. Craven, a general practitioner at Glendale Memorial Hospital, California. His hypothesis was based on the fact that a heart attack was due to thrombus formation and that aspirin could prevent clot formation. In 1948, he prescribed aspirin to 400 patients and reported, in 1950, that none of them had suffered a heart attack during the two-year period. He made another keen observation: patients who underwent surgery for the removal of tonsils had continued bleeding if they chewed aspirin gum for pain relief, a phenomenon he had never seen before in his thirty years of carrying out tonsil surgeries. To further support his idea that aspirin prevented clotting and promoted bleeding, he stated that men were more likely to suffer from heart attacks than women because they were less likely to take aspirin for common aches and pains. He prescribed aspirin to men between the ages of forty-five and sixty-five who were overweight and led sedentary lives. In a follow-up paper in 1953, he reported that none of his 1,500 patients who faithfully took the drug suffered a heart attack. Craven acknowledged the limitations of his study but stated that the results had given some 'preliminary impressions' that might be substantiated or refuted by subsequent research.

Craven wasn't just content with observational studies—he personally took twelve aspirin tablets daily for five days, which resulted in spontaneous nose bleeding. He repeated the experiment twice over with precisely the same results. The fact that he hadn't had a nosebleed in fifty years added value to his experiment. In 1956, he published another paper, updating the results of his trial. He had put 8,000 patients on aspirin prophylaxis, out of which only nine had died of heart attacks. Upon autopsy, the cause of death in these patients was not thrombus but ruptured arteries. In the same paper, he also highlighted the role of aspirin in the prevention of 'little strokes' (transient ischemic attacks), for none of his patients suffered one.

In the late 1960s, Harvey J. Weiss began his experiments on the effects of aspirin on platelet aggregation. His research concluded that low doses of aspirin prevented platelet aggregation by inhibiting the release of the molecule ADP. He also proved that the acetyl group of aspirin was crucial for this inhibition and that the effect was irreversible.

In 1971, John Vane, professor of pharmacology at the University of London, published his research on the inhibition of prostaglandin synthesis by aspirin. He was awarded the Nobel Prize for his work in 1982.

Today, aspirin is used widely as a pain killer and as an anti-inflammatory drug. It is also used for the prevention of heart attacks and strokes due to its antiplatelet action. Recent research has even hinted at its potential to prevent cancers of the colon.

7

Clot Busters and Retrievers

Serendipity is not the product of patience; it's the product of action.

—Audrey Moralez

IN HIS BOOK *The Serendipity Mindset*, Dr Christian Busch describes three different types of serendipity.

Archimedes serendipity: An unexpected way to solve the problem we wanted to solve. This occurs when a known problem or challenge is solved but the solution comes from an unexpected source. The Greek mathematician Archimedes exemplified this when he was trying to determine if a goldsmith has substituted silver for gold in a crown meant for the king. Archimedes stumbled upon the solution during a bath, when he saw the water level rise as he entered the tub. He realized that a crown mixed with silver, which is lighter than gold, would have to be bulkier to weigh the same. Therefore, when submerged in water, it would displace more water than a pure gold crown of the same weight.

Post-it note serendipity: An unexpected solution to a different problem from the one you originally wanted to solve. This occurs when you examine a particular problem but stumble across a solution to an entirely different or previously unrecognized problem. In the late 1970s, Dr Spencer Silver, a researcher at the consumer goods company 3M, was trying to concoct a stronger glue. Instead, he derived a substance that didn't stick particularly well. But this glue turned out to be perfect for a new product line that 3M called Post-it notes.

Thunderbolt serendipity: An effortless solution to an unexpected or unrealized problem. This occurs when there is no problem-solving underway. It is entirely unexpected, like a thunderbolt from a clear sky, and sparks a new opportunity or solves a previously unknown or unattempted problem. Many new ideas and approaches emerge from this type of serendipity.

All the above examples of serendipity are very interesting. The common theme amongst them all is 'unexpected'. We are often presented with opportunities unexpectedly, and it is then upon us to turn them into positive outcomes. We have seen how the potential of aspirin as an antiplatelet agent was recognized and now it is widely used for the prevention of strokes and heart attacks. This chapter also focuses on how we unexpectedly got hold of drugs that caused a revolution in stroke care.

The search for antibiotics in the 1930s, the discovery of the double-helix structure of DNA and an extremely aggressive case of melanoma skin cancer in the 1970s together contributed to a breakthrough treatment for heart attacks and ischemic stroke. Unrelated areas of research unexpectedly converged and unsuccessful experiments in one area led to sudden advances in another.

During my internship in India, a few years ago, I attended to many patients coming to the emergency room with chest pain and breathlessness. A heart attack, or myocardial infarction (MI), is basically a blockage, usually by a clot, in one of the arteries supplying blood to the heart, causing damage to the heart muscle and thus impeding the effective pumping of blood. On such occasions, our immediate response was to give the patient oxygen and call for an ECG. A cardiologist would then diagnose the MI from the ECG results and discuss treatment options with the patient's family. There were two main choices to dissolve the clot: a more affordable injection, priced at Rs 4,000, and an expensive one, coming in at Rs 40,000. The cheaper option, streptokinase, had various side effects, such as the increased risk of internal bleeding or severe allergic reactions. The more expensive alternative was rtPA. For ischemic stroke patients, however, streptokinase was not even an option due to its very high risk of bleeding, leaving rtPA as the sole remedy.

STREPTOKINASE

In the 1930s, bacterial infections were a major public health concern. In pursuing antibiotics, researchers were studying bacteria called streptococci to understand the disease process and to find ways to subdue infections. Whenever there is an infection, the body tries to contain it by laying down a fibrin-like substance around it. But certain bacteria, like streptococcus, the 'flesh-eating bacteria', have mechanisms to break down that barrier and spread to deeper and deeper layers of tissue, causing conditions like cellulitis.

The drug streptokinase was discovered through sheer serendipity. Dr William Smith Tillett, associate professor of medicine and director of the biological division at Johns Hopkins University, made a noteworthy observation in 1933: streptococci agglutinated (clumped together) in test tubes containing human plasma but not in those that contained human serum. Plasma is the fluid (devoid of blood cells) part of the blood that contains clotting factors, while serum does not contain clotting factors. Where most people would have dismissed this as trivial, Tillett considered it significant. He inferred that agglutination of streptococci is caused by a component of plasma that is deficient in serum. The primary candidate was fibrinogen, a key clotting factor. He hypothesized that fibrinogen was adsorbed on the surface of streptococci, which led to the clumping of the bacteria. Tillett theorized that if the bacteria in the plasma used up the fibrinogen, then a sample of plasma containing streptococci would not clot.

In order to prove his hypothesis, he took five test tubes containing human plasma and added streptococci, leaving the other three as controls. He was hoping that streptococci would adsorb the fibrinogen and prevent clot formation. However, to his dismay, the results of this experiment were uniformly negative: there was clot formation in all the test tubes, regardless of the presence of streptococci.

Disheartened, Tillet left the test tubes in the rack without bothering to clean them. However, he continued to wonder what could have gone wrong with his assumption that had seemed so plausible. Drawn back to his test tubes one last time before discarding them, he observed, to his delight, that there was free liquid in the subset of the test tubes containing the streptococcal cultures. The bacteria had not prevented clot formation by using up the fibrin but had instead broken down the clot after it was formed. This led him to conclude that the streptococci had synthesized a fibrinolytic agent that was responsible for dissolving the clots. This was the probable mechanism for clot lysis (break down), rather than adsorption of fibrinogen, as he had earlier presumed. He called this substance fibrinolysin (later christened streptokinase) and managed to isolate the protein in its stable form with his colleague R.L. Garner.

Consider what happens when we get a paper cut: there is a little bleeding, then the blood clots and within a few days the cut seals up completely. The blood clot is a temporary seal, and the body has mechanisms to dissolve it and replace it with new skin. The substance that dissolves blood clots in the body is plasmin. Plasmin exists in blood in an inactive form (just like the clotting factors from the sticker analogy in the previous chapter). The inactive form of plasmin is called plasminogen. This plasminogen is converted into the clot-dissolving plasmin by the tissue plasminogen activator (tPA) present in the body. All these factors work in a synchronous fashion in the body, such that when the clot needs to be formed, these clot-dissolving factors are inactive and vice versa. It was discovered that streptokinase converted plasminogen into its active form, plasmin, which lysed clots.

In 1947, Tillet appointed Sol Sherry to investigate the clinical potential of streptokinase. They chose cases of haemothorax (blood around the lungs) and empyema (pus around the lungs), because in these particular cases the effects could be easily seen on radiographs and the fluid could be drawn for analysis. They injected streptokinase into the chest of a patient with loculated haemothorax and found that all the loculations dissolved within six hours. After extraction of the lysed coagulum, chest X-rays showed the pleural space drained of its previous contents.

This streptokinase preparation was only 10 per cent pure. It contained other enzymes and caused various side effects, such as fever, malaise, joint pains and occasional nausea. It was not suitable to be injected into the bloodstream. Lederle Laboratories, in 1957, successfully developed purified preparations of streptokinase, which were tolerated well by patients. The next year, Sol Sherry and his colleagues reported the first study of intravenously administered streptokinase in patients with acute myocardial infarction. They demonstrated that patients treated within fourteen hours had lower in-hospital mortality rates, while the ones treated anywhere between twenty and seventy-two hours had mortality rates akin to those of untreated patients, thus highlighting the need for early intervention.

However, the role of thrombolytic therapy was not readily accepted, instead going on to be heavily debated for decades. This was because some cardiologists, such as William C. Roberts, suggested that coronary thrombosis was a 'result', rather than a 'cause' of myocardial necrosis (heart muscle damage). They pointed to abnormal ECG readings suggestive of heart muscle spasms and noted that about one-third of patients had no post-mortem clots (though this was because the body's natural fibrinolytic system had dissolved them).

A shift in perception occurred in 1980, when Marcus DeWood and his colleagues published a landmark paper in Spokane, Washington. They performed coronary angiography (then considered to be a dangerous procedure) in live patients within twenty-four hours of onset of symptoms. Their findings were revelatory: out of 126 patients, 110 exhibited coronary blockage. In half of these patients, clots were retrieved using a Fogarty catheter. This led to a resurgence of thrombolytic therapy for myocardial infarction. Similarly, with the advent of pulmonary angiography, urokinase (isolated from human urine) and streptokinase were used for clot lysis of pulmonary emboli.

However, thrombolytic therapy with streptokinase for ischemic stroke turned out to be more detrimental than beneficial due to the risk of severe bleeding. Many trials were, in fact, terminated due to the serious adverse effects. This was because streptokinase not only activated the plasminogen bound to the fibrin clot but also activated it systemically, producing plasmin, which degraded various molecules involved in the coagulation cascade and predisposed other organs to bleeding.

In the early 1960s, a group led by the neurologist John S. Meyer at Wayne State University performed several studies on the efficacy of thrombolytic therapy with outcomes ranging from uncertain to bad to worse. In one cohort of seventy-three patients, Meyer reported that thirteen of the thirty-seven patients who received streptokinase died, in stark contrast to the four deaths observed among the thirty-six control subjects.

tPA

Tissue plasminogen activator, or tPA, as previously discussed, is the substance present in the body that converts plasminogen into plasmin. tPA was first discovered in 1947 by Danish investigators Tage Astrup and Per M. Permin. They observed that when clots were introduced into slices of tissues taken from various mammals, such as oxen, pigs, rabbits and rats, they dissolved.

The agent responsible was thought to be tPA. Scientists were, however, unable to separate tPA from the tissues in which it was found. It resisted purification. Making a drug out of tPA was thus inconceivable due to its scarcity. Between the detection of tPA and its availability in purified form, thirty-five years would elapse.

Cells in the body grow and divide to produce more cells, but the process of division is strictly controlled. When cells divide incessantly and produce more and more cells, they can cause cancer. Aggressive cancers grow and spread rapidly, invading more and more tissue. This is due to their ability to produce enzymes that break down normal tissue structures and boundaries. These enzymes work like plasmin, the clot-dissolving enzyme.

Like all systems and enzymes in the body, plasmin's actions are closely regulated. Hence, the body has certain inhibitors to its actions, which prevent premature clot lysis. One such inhibitor is alpha 2-antiplasmin. In 1974, Belgian researcher Désiré Collen was working to use its potential to stop the growth and spread of cancer cells. Collen was trained both as a biochemist and a physician. He ran a multidisciplinary laboratory and forged close relationships with researchers in many fields, both in Europe and the United States.

In 1978, Collen was visited by Daniel B. Rifkin, a cell biologist at the Rockefeller University. Rifkin, who had been studying tumour development, was working on the Bowes melanoma cell line, named after the patient from whom it originated. This aggressive cell line produced large amounts of a protease causing fibrinolysis (an enzyme that broke down fibrin). In a mutual exchange, Rifkin gave Collen the cell line, while Collen gave him some of the anti-plasmin. Collen then began investigating the substance produced by the Bowes cell line but was initially unable to extract and purify it. He conducted a series of experiments and found that the substance had a very high affinity for fibrin present in the clot.

The following year, Dingeman Rijken, who had previously worked on tPA, joined Collen's laboratory. Rijken had earlier managed to recover a minuscule amount of tPA from uterine tissue. The trick to purification turned out to be a simple detergent, widely known to chemists as Tween 80. Applied to the Bowes extract, it worked like a charm. Within a month, Collen and Rijken could say with confidence that this substance—they were still calling it melanoma plasminogen activator at the time—was homogenous and that it could not be distinguished, by any known assay or test, from tPA.

Collen now attempted to scale up production, but it was never enough. Over the next couple of years, his laboratory managed to produce a bit more than half a teaspoonful. Though it was a tiny amount, it was enough for substantive research and even a few clinical applications.

After various experiments, Collen and Rijken established that tPA dissolved pulmonary emboli in rabbits and treated coronary artery thrombosis in experimental dogs. The first human to be treated was a thirty-year-old woman who had undergone a kidney transplant and was suffering from the complication of renal vein thrombosis. The clot could be seen floating in the inferior vena cava upon X-ray examination. When the treating physician, Willem Weimar, injected the patient with tPA provided by Collen, the clot completely dissolved, leaving no side effects.

Although the two grams of tPA produced by Collen and his colleagues represented a thousand times more than what had been produced over the course of more than three decades, it was insignificant in pharmaceutical terms. The Bowes cell line itself was an unlikely source.

The solution came from biotechnology, an alliance of biochemistry and molecular engineering. The biotech industry uses bacteria and other organisms to manufacture biological products in large quantities. An early biotech avatar was the company Genentech. In 1973, a few years before the company was founded, one of its founders, Herb Boyer, together with fellow researcher Stanley Cohen, first demonstrated what became known as recombinant genetic engineering. They extracted DNA from the African clawed frog and made multiple copies of a specific DNA sequence. They integrated this DNA with the bacteria E. coli. The idea was that this process could compel bacteria, which divide in minutes and multiply exponentially, to fabricate ample amounts of peptides and proteins as the basis for useful drugs. Persuaded by the head of research management at Stanford University, Boyer and Cohen applied for a patent in 1974, which was eventually granted. Meanwhile, after Boyer and entrepreneur Robert Swanson created a partnership, Genentech was born in San Francisco in 1976.

A year later, in 1977, the company produced the first synthetic protein, somatostatin, and two years later managed to clone it. The journey to clinical application, however, was not immediate. Genentech scientists also won the scientific race to clone the human gene for insulin, used to treat diabetes. Synthetic insulin would eventually replace insulin harvested from the organs of cows, to which some patients developed allergies. Business advanced apace, and in 1980, Genentech aroused much interest on Wall Street, when its stock price leapt from $35 to $88 the day of its initial public offering. Genentech developed an aggressive legal strategy to patent and protect every single one of its molecular products, and within twenty years it held more than 7,500 patents, granted or pending.

tPA soon became a candidate for Genentech's portfolio. Like both insulin and somatostatin, it was the product of a single, large gene. However, where recombinant insulin would simply replace an animal analogue and somatostatin would be used to treat a relatively uncommon condition, tPA was poised to be a genuinely novel drug for major disorders like heart attacks, which in 1980, occurred on average once every twenty seconds, resulting in 588 deaths per 100,000 people annually in the United States. The potential for addressing strokes, though not yet a primary focus, was also significant.

Genentech's decision to find out more about tPA was due to Herb Heyneker, a Dutch biochemist, one of the original Genentech scientists and later a businessman. While reading the literature on urokinase, which Genentech had contracted to clone just because tiny amounts of it already existed, he stumbled upon tPA. Now, he learnt, it too was extracted and purified. Heyneker immediately recognized the potential and told colleagues that it 'sounds even more interesting than urokinase'.

In 1980, Heyneker sent Diane Pennica, a newly hired young PhD, to a European congress on fibrinolysis, where Collen would present his findings. Pennica arrived early in Malmo, Sweden, introduced herself to Collen and explained why she was there. Collen invited her to join him and other investigators for dinner. It was there that she suggested cloning tPA and convinced Collen to supply the purified tPA/melanoma protein under a contractual agreement.

Today, cloning a gene of 2,530 base pairs of DNA for a protein that consists of 527 amino acids would be largely automated and take a few days at most. This was not the case in 1980. The process was one of painstaking reverse engineering. The long chains of amino acids that make up the protein had to be deconstructed and back-translated into the genetic code embedded in the nucleotide sequences of DNA. The unique gene itself had to be sought within the genome and sequenced in its entirety. After about six months, Pennica's laboratory produced a single, incomplete match between a short DNA sequence and a series of amino acids in a fragment of tPA. Another half-year's work and the full sequence was worked out. Pennica and her group confirmed that the human genome contains a single gene that codes for tPA, provided its complete sequence and structure, and demonstrated that it performed as promised. She presented her results at the sixth International Congress on Fibrinolysis in Lausanne, Switzerland, in July 1982, and her paper was published in the science journal *Nature* the following January.

This crucial research paved the way for the development of recombinant tPA (rtPA).

THROMBECTOMY

An ischemic stroke is similar to a clogged water pipe. A water pipe can get clogged due to hard water, which contains various minerals that can precipitate and clog the pipe. You can prevent this by installing a water softener. Similarly, one can prevent the formation of clots that block blood vessels by using blood thinners, as we discussed in the previous chapters. Once the pipe gets clogged, you can clean it with drain cleaners and chemicals or a plumber can mechanically pull out the material blocking the pipe. Similarly, tPA is the chemical that can dissolve the clots blocking the blood vessels. In certain situations, such as when a patient has contradictions to the use of tPA or when the clot is too big or in a very vital blood vessel, neuro-interventionalists can use catheters to reach the blocked blood vessels and mechanically remove the clots. In some patients, more than one of the two approaches can be combined.

Over the past decade, catheter-based mechanical thrombectomy (*ectomy* meaning 'removal') techniques to reopen acutely occluded arteries have seen rapid technical advancements. The devices can either fish out the clot (retrieval devices) or suck it out (aspiration devices). Mechanical techniques have several advantages over clot-dissolving drugs. They work more rapidly, achieving recanalization by opening the blood vessel within a few minutes, compared to the 120 minutes required with lytic drug administration. They also pose a reduced risk of brain haemorrhage or systemic haemorrhage. They are more effective in removing large clot burdens, where the sheer volume to be digested impedes pharmacological lysis.

Suction thrombectomy devices use vacuum aspiration to suck the occlusive clot out of the blocked artery. The first successful suction device was the Penumbra system. The evolution of aspiration devices had to address the issue of aspiration tips becoming blocked, a common occurrence when applying suction through the small catheter tubes that could be manoeuvred to intracranial arteries. The Penumbra system overcame this obstacle by adding a separator wire with a bulbous tip inside the suction tube. As the vacuum operates, the physician continually advances and retracts the separator wire, keeping the tip of the tube clear and also pulling in the thrombus ahead of the catheter.

A recent innovation in suction thrombectomy has been the development of large bore catheters. These are both flexible and manoeuvrable enough to target clots in the intracranial arteries. With these larger devices, clogging isn't an issue during direct aspiration, even without a separator wire. Moreover, substantial vacuum power can be generated simply by having the physician pull back strongly with a syringe.

Clot retrieval devices were first developed to capture coils and other foreign bodies that had embolized within the brain circulation during other endovascular procedures, such as aneurysmal coiling (we'll discuss this in Chapter 9). A natural next step was to apply these devices to capture and remove naturally arising thromboemboli. These devices ensnare a thrombus and then withdraw it out of the body. The first approved family of retrieval devices were the MERCI retrievers, which operate much like corkscrews, and pull the clot out of the artery in a manner similar to removing the cork from a wine bottle. The Mechanical Embolus Removal in Cerebral Ischemia (MERCI) study evaluated the safety and efficacy of this mechanical embolectomy device. As a result of this trial, the MERCI retriever, in 2004, became the first device approved by the US FDA for use in patients with acute intracranial occlusions.

The most recent and most successful family of thrombectomy devices to be developed are the stent retrievers. These are mesh columns that are expanded inside the target clot, pushing it aside and entangling it within the crossing struts of the stents. The stent is then withdrawn in its unfolded state, bringing out with it the enmeshed thrombus. Stent retrievers have two major advantages over MERCI corkscrews and other retrieval devices. Firstly, there is an immediate restoration of blood flow upon deployment within the target artery, rather than only upon successful clot extraction. Secondly, the rates of recanalization are substantially higher than that of other embolectomy devices.

8

Imaging

One such shortcoming is that structures in three-dimensional space overlap in a conventional, two-dimensional X-ray photograph. What we see is a shadow play—a play, alas, with far too many actors on the stage. It becomes difficult to discern the villain ... Ordinary X-ray examinations of the head had shown the skull bones, but the brain had remained a gray, undifferentiated fog. Now, suddenly, the fog had cleared.

—Nobel Prize Committee (on the discovery of the CT scan), 1979

If you want to find the secrets of the universe, think in terms of energy, frequency and vibration.

—Nikola Tesla

IN THE PAST, stroke diagnoses often occurred at autopsies. Neuropathologists would dissect the brain, examining its slices to determine the cause of death. We currently have technology that can show us the inside of the brain without cutting it open, and in a matter of minutes. Doctors can now safely and quickly discern whether a patient's stroke is due to a haemorrhage or an ischemia. The two most commonly used brain scans are the CT scan and the MRI. On a CT scan, a haemorrhage appears white, whereas infarcts (dead tissue due to an ischemic stroke) appear grey or black, making it quite easy to distinguish the two main stroke categories. There are a number of different types of images that can be obtained using an MRI: Some MRI sequences effectively show areas of infarction even minutes after they develop, while others best show areas of bleeding.

Brain scans not only show whether the lesion is haemorrhagic or ischemic, but they also show where the abnormality is located, how large and extensive it is, and whether there is brain swelling and pressure inside the head caused by the infarct or haemorrhage. Upon spotting stroke-related abnormalities, doctors then test the arteries that supply the injured brain. Pictures of the arteries (angiograms) can be created using a CT scanner. An iodine-containing dye is injected into the patient and then rapid pictures are taken as it travels through the brain's arteries and veins. These are called CT angiograms and can be obtained at the same time as a CT scan. Alternatively, magnetic resonance angiograms (MRA) can be made without injecting the dye. Blood moving through the arteries and veins will appear in the image if the settings on the MRI machine are made to capture these vascular structures instead of the brain.

Ultrasound, sometimes called Doppler ultrasound in honour of the physicist Christian Doppler, is another effective and safe way to study arterial blood flow. During this procedure, a small probe is placed over blood vessels in the neck, as well as over the eyes and the back and sides of the head. The probe gathers ultrasound information, which is processed by an analysing machine that creates pictures of the vessels and also calculates the speed of the blood moving through the blood vessels directly under the probes. Ultrasound findings can tell us if an artery is normal, narrowed or completely blocked.

When these three non-invasive tests do not provide sufficient information, physicians may order a digital subtraction angiogram (DSA). In this procedure, a catheter is inserted through the peripheral arteries (such as the arteries in the groin or the arm) and is advanced to the arteries in the brain. A contrast material is then injected into those arteries. An image (known as a mask image) of the region is taken before injecting the contrast material. As this contrast material travels through the blood vessels, contrast images are taken in succession. These images show the opacified arteries superimposed on the mask image and are stored on the computer. The mask image is then subtracted from the contrast images, pixel by pixel. The resulting subtraction images show only the filled vessels. These pictures of the inside of the arteries display areas of narrowing or blockage, aneurysms and vascular malformations. Occasionally, during the DSA, the specialist may proceed with treatments to open narrowed or blocked arteries (the clot retrieval discussed in Chapter 7) or to obliterate vascular malformations or aneurysms (coiling, which will be discussed in Chapter 9).

CEREBRAL ANGIOGRAPHY

António Egas Moniz was born on 29 November 1874 in the village of Avança, Northern Portugal. He joined the University of Coimbra at the age of seventeen to study mathematics. He then decided to pursue medicine, and in 1899, at the age of twenty-five, received his bachelor's degree. In 1901, he earned his Doctor of Medicine degree, and later joined the University of Coimbra as a lecturer. Egas Moniz travelled regularly to France and trained with some of the country's leading neurologists, such as Joseph Babinski and Jean-Athanase Sicard. In 1911, he moved to Lisbon to join the University of Lisbon as a professor of neurology. He was also active in politics and was elected as a member of parliament in 1903, going on to become the minister of foreign affairs in 1917. At the same time, he was a prolific writer, publishing several books, articles and biographies. He was fond of art and playing cards and even wrote on the origin of the latter. In 1919, he retired from politics and committed himself to neurological research.

When Egas Moniz re-entered the field of neurology, the only method available to visualize and diagnose brain tumours was pneumoencephalography (*pneumato*, meaning 'air' and *encephalo*, meaning 'relating to the brain'). It was a gruesome procedure in which the cerebrospinal fluid surrounding the brain was drained and replaced by air, oxygen or helium to present a better contrast between the brain and its crevices on X-rays. It was an extremely painful procedure for the patient: they would be strapped to a chair and rotated to different positions, even upside down, causing various side effects, such as headache, vomiting, increased heart rate, neck stiffness and confusion.

Egas Moniz was inspired by Jean-Athanase Sicard's technique of visualizing the lesions of the spinal cord by injecting lipiodol as a contrast material into the cerebrospinal fluid. He began working on a method to visualize brain tumours by injecting radio-opaque materials into the arteries. He called this technique *encéphalographie artérielle* (arterial encephalography), for it would visualize the blood vessels. He then began looking for a suitable material that would provide a good contrast without blocking the arteries. Lipiodol wasn't suitable for the blood vessels and would also cause serious side effects. Egas Moniz therefore conducted his experiments using strontium bromide, lithium bromide and sodium iodide on cadavers, dogs, rabbits and, finally, humans. The autopsy material for his studies was not readily available, so he began transporting decapitated heads of corpses in boxes from the Anatomical Institute to his laboratory in his Cadillac. He obtained excellent radiographs (X-rays) with the contrast material in cadaver heads.

Egas Moniz initially attempted to achieve results in humans by administering bromides orally, but he obtained no radiograms. He then tried injecting strontium bromide subcutaneously (under the skin) and obtained two non-diagnostic films and one that was barely detectable. In one of the cases, the vessel got ruptured and the contrast spread to the surrounding tissues. He concluded that the failure of the experiment was due to the very thin size of the needles, which would have easily dislodged from the vessels. In his next set of experiments, the internal carotid arteries were opened surgically, and after occluding the proximal segment, the dye was injected into them. The arteries were visualized in one of the patients, but he died eight hours later due to thrombosis, as the dye was too dense to allow blood flow. Disheartened, Egas Moniz discontinued his research for a while.

However, upon discussions with his collaborator and friend Almeida Lima, he decided to continue his experiments by replacing strontium bromide with sodium iodide as the contrast. It was on 28 June 1927 that they finally obtained the first arteriogram of a twenty-year-old patient, which displayed a huge pituitary tumour. Egas Moniz presented his discovery at the congress of the Neurological Society in Paris and was extolled by renowned neurologists like Babinski, Sicard and Clovis Vincent. The contrast material sodium iodide was further replaced by thorotrast. Egas Moniz began publishing various articles on the applications of cerebral angiography and on internal carotid artery occlusion. It is interesting to note that, despite his integral role in these advances, Egas Moniz never conducted a single intervention himself, for his hands were severely deformed by gout. They were instead conducted by Lima, who later became a neurosurgeon.

Though Egas Moniz was nominated thrice for the Nobel Prize for the invention of cerebral angiography, he was rejected all three times. The first rejection cited the limited number of cases on whom the procedure was performed, while subsequent rejections were because the committee believed that ventriculography (pneumoencephalography) had contributed much more to the field.

In 1949, Egas Moniz became the first Portuguese citizen to be awarded the Nobel Prize in Physiology or Medicine. However, this wasn't for his discovery of cerebral angiography but for the discovery of leucotomy, a form of psychosurgery. Egas Moniz believed that several mental illnesses, including schizophrenia, could be cured by severing the white matter connections in the brain. Initially, he tried achieving this by using alcohol injections. When this failed, he devised the leucotome, an instrument comprising a hollow needle with an embedded blade. It was introduced through a hole in the skull into the white matter and was rotated to cut out a 1-cm sphere. The first procedure was performed by Almeida Lima, assisted by Ruy Lacerada.

The procedure became widespread after its adoption by Walter Freeman, who himself performed around 3,000 leucotomies. Freeman also operated on Rosemary Kennedy, John F. Kennedy's sister, though this had devastating consequences that left her incapable of living independently. The procedure fell into disrepute and faced widespread protests. As written by Francisco González-Crussi in his book *A Short History of Medicine*:

> What was once hailed by the media as a momentous medical breakthrough, a fast clean way that 'surgical wizardry' had discovered to restore sanctity to the severely disturbed, was now exposed for what it really was: a reckless, irreversible mutilation inflicted on people based on an overly simplistic conception of the working of the human mind.

The irony here is clear: leucotomy, later condemned, earned Egas Moniz the Nobel Prize, while cerebral angiography, an important diagnostic tool, was rejected for the Nobel Prize on three occasions.

The cerebral angiography technique developed by Moniz involved the injection of a dye in the artery of the neck by directly puncturing the vessel through the skin. This was a very invasive procedure and risky too, since it involved puncturing a large vessel which could cause significant bleeding. Currently, the conventional technique developed by Moniz is not used. The modern approach is digital subtraction angiography as discussed above.

In 1953, Sven Ivar Seldinger, a pioneering Swedish interventional radiologist working at the Karolinska Hospital, introduced a novel method of gaining vascular access, employing a hollow needle, an exchange wire and a catheter. His technique enabled radiologists to perform angiographies in a relatively risk-free manner by puncturing smaller vessels in the arm or the groin and then advancing catheters to the other vessels in the body. This led to the emergence of minimally invasive procedures. Today, this method forms the foundation of a number of procedures, such as digital subtraction angiography and the insertion of central venous catheters, chest drains and pacemakers.

It was by building on the work of Seldinger that Charles Dotter and Andreas Gruentzig developed angioplasty.

ᶜ∕ᵒ

CT SCAN

Traditional X-rays struggled to image the brain. The skull's radio density and the fluid surrounding the brain made it appear as a homogenous density without any details of its structure (what the quote at the start of this chapter describes as 'a gray, undifferentiated fog'). Cerebral angiography too had certain risks associated with the dye, and it was an invasive procedure, involving the artery being punctured. Thus, the pursuit of finding a non-invasive modality continued.

The solution came in the form of the CT scan, an innovation that earned Allan M. Cormack and Godfrey N. Hounsfield the Nobel Prize in Physiology or Medicine in 1979. Remarkably, neither was a medical doctor, and both pursued independent research, completely unaware of each other's work.

Allan M. Cormack was a nuclear physicist at the University of Cape Town. When the hospital physicist resigned, he was asked to supervise the radioactive isotope doses for cancer therapy at Groote Schuur Hospital. He realized that the method used for calculation was imprecise and was developed considering the body to be a homogenous media. His primary aim was thus to calculate the radiation attenuation coefficients of different parts of the body for better treatment. Understanding that the problem was primarily mathematical, he formulated equations and conducted various experiments to reconstruct an accurate cross-section of an irregularly shaped object. He reported his findings in two articles published in 1963 and 1964. Using a simple desktop calculator as his 'computer', he produced the first computerized tomograms ever made. He was aware of the potential of his method to produce X-ray or positron camera images of cross-sectional slices of the body. However, the computers of his time were not capable of executing the enormous calculations that the procedure required. Hence, no apparatus of practical diagnostic importance was constructed.

The Beatles, the best-selling and arguably the most influential band in music history, signed with Electric and Music Industries Ltd (EMI) in 1962. The band was an almost immediate hit, and EMI earned millions of dollars through them—so much so that it didn't know what to do with that level of revenue. One beneficiary was a scientist working with the company, Godfrey Hounsfield, who led the team that built the first all-transistor computer in 1958. EMI gave Hounsfield the freedom to conduct independent research and funded it with the profits made by the Beatles. Thus, the Beatles indirectly contributed to the development of the CT scan.

Hounsfield's idea was to take multiple radiographic images of an object and reconstruct it by using a computerized technique.

The first prototype of the machine made by Hounsfield consisted of a gamma ray radiation source, for he couldn't afford an X-ray source. The radiation source was placed in a lead box with a pinhole, through which a single beam of radiation was projected onto the object and recorded on a detector on the opposite side. This was placed on a lathe bed and the beam was moved across the entire object. The disk under the object was then rotated by one degree and the beam was passed again. This process was repeated till a rotation of 180 degrees was achieved. Hounsfield took around 28,000 measurements, digitized them and recorded them on paper tape. The gamma source used, however, was extremely slow, and the machine had to operate for nine days straight to get the image. The computer then took another two and a half hours to process the data and produce the image.

Recognizing these limitations, Hounsfield shifted to an X-ray tube, which gave a more detailed image in a shorter span of time—about nine hours. The first image was of an animal brain, showing grey and white matter. He realized that the formalin used to preserve the specimen was enhancing the image, leading to exaggerated results. He then experimented with fresh bullocks' brains, but the ventricles of those brains were filled with blood, due to the method used during slaughter, so no satisfactory images were procured. His pursuit of optimal samples led him to Jewish kosher houses in London, where he found animals who had been drained of their blood before being slaughtered. These were perfect specimens for imaging.

After getting satisfactory results with animal brains, Hounsfield built an improved prototype for clinical use. The first scanner, dubbed the EMI Mark I, was installed at Atkinson Morley Hospital in Wimbledon. The apparatus was primarily designed to image the brain and had a small opening just for the head. The first tomographic examination took place on 1 October 1971, and was of a woman with a suspected brain tumour. A cystic lesion in the frontal lobe was easily distinguished, for it was much darker than the surrounding healthy tissue. The scan took about four and a half minutes, and the image was reconstructed in about twenty seconds. The scan was witnessed by the neurologists James Ambrose and Louis Kreel. Hounsfield presented his results at a seminar at the British Institute of Radiology in April 1972 and published his findings in various journals, including the *British Journal of Radiology*. EMI, however, could not keep up with the mass production of CT scanners, so this was subsequently taken up by other technological giants.

Hounsfield continued to work on modifying the scanners. Faster scanning systems led to the development of complete body scanners, which could image constantly moving organs like the heart and the lungs. The first full body scan was taken of Hounsfield himself. In addition to the Nobel Prize, Hounsfield received many other awards and was appointed Commander of the Order of the British Empire in 1976 and was knighted five years later. The Hounsfield scale is used as a measurement tool for radiodensity even today. Beyond CT technology, Hounsfield made contributions to the development of MRI as well.

First-generation scanners consisted of a single radiation beam and a single detector, which had a translation motion across the object followed by a rotation by a degree and another translation motion, till it completed 180 degrees. Second-generation scanners used a fan beam instead of a single beam and multiple detectors. The third generation had a row of fixed multiple detectors forming a complete circle, which remained stationary while the beam moved. The earlier models could rotate only 180 degrees, as the wires in the circuit would entangle otherwise. With the development of slip ring technology, helical scanners were developed, which could rotate 360 degrees. As these modern scanners complete one rotation, the patient is moved through it, giving a resultant helical motion.

Today's CT scanners function at tremendous speeds, enabling a full-body scan in less than a minute. With advancements in technology, innovations such as contrast-enhanced computed tomography (CECT) and high-resolution computed tomography (HRCT) have come up.

The CT scan is an indispensable tool in the fields of neurology and neurosurgery. A haemorrhagic stroke can easily be distinguished from an ischemic one on a CT scan. In fact, the precise location and the severity of a bleed can be identified. As trauma victims are brought to the emergency room, they are evaluated to rule out brain or cervical spine injuries through a CT scan. The progression of a disease process can be easily observed, and treatments can be modified accordingly. Unnecessary neurosurgical interventions can be avoided in certain conditions and the patient can be treated conservatively. It can also distinguish tumours and degenerative lesions of the brain. Metaphorically speaking, the CT scan is a window into the skull, providing an unprecedented view of its workings.

MRI

Raymond Damadian always believed that while a medical practitioner could impact thousands of lives, a researcher could impact millions. After completing an undergraduate degree in chemistry, he studied at the Albert Einstein College of Medicine. He followed this with an internship and residency in internal medicine at SUNY Downstate Medical Center in Brooklyn. Damadian was fascinated by how the kidneys maintain the proper electrical state of the body by balancing the electrically active sodium and potassium ions. So, after his residency, he worked as a postdoctoral fellow in nephrology. During this time, Dr Freeman Winder Cope of Pennsylvania asked Damadian to collaborate with him and study how potassium ions were accumulated in the cells of the body using the new nuclear magnetic resonance (NMR) technology for chemical analysis. Damadian managed to arrange a bacterium from the Dead Sea, *Halobacter halobium*, which possessed about twenty times more potassium than was found in normal cells. Freeman put the bacteria in a test tube, wrapped an antenna around the test tube and put it in the NMR machine. He measured the exact amount of K^+ ions in that cell of the bacterium within seconds using the NMR. This fascinated Damadian, given the time-intensive nature of conventional chemical analyses and led him to consider using the NMR to detect the differences between normal and cancerous tissues.

The phenomenon of nuclear magnetic resonance (NMR) was discovered by Isidor I. Rabi, a Columbia University physics professor in 1937. Rabi recognized that atomic nuclei show their presence by absorbing or emitting radio waves exposed to a strong magnetic field. Felix Bloch and Edward Purcell received the Nobel Prize for Physics in 1952 for demonstrating how atomic nuclei in a magnetic field absorb and re-emit electromagnetic radiation. What we now know as magnetic resonance imaging, or MRI, originated from NMR technology. The prefix 'N', for nuclear, was dropped since it implied radioactivity, which the MRI did not actually use. The 'I', for imaging, was added by the medical community to identify MR as an imaging technology.

Damadian's next step was to acquire rats bearing Walker sarcoma tumours. He excised the tumour and put the sample in the NMR machine to compare the NMR signals with that of normal tissues. He found them to be dramatically different. He confirmed his findings by experimenting on rats containing other types of tumours, going on to publish a paper titled 'Tumour Detection by Nuclear Magnetic Resonance' in the 19 March 1971 issue of the magazine *Science*. Now, the challenge for him was to convert the small test-tube scanner into a full-sized scanner of the human body.

Paul Lauterbur held a PhD in NMR and was the co-founder of the company NMR Specialities, headquartered in New Kensington, Pennsylvania. NMR Specialities made its equipment available to potential customers as a sales strategy. On 2 September 1971, Leon Saryan, a post-doctoral fellow at Johns Hopkins, came to NMR Specialities in order to confirm the findings of Raymond Damadian's *Science* paper. Lauterbur observed Saryan's experiment and noticed the differences between the signals of normal and malignant tissue. Saryan brought samples cut out from rats. Lauterbur, being a chemist, was not used to such cuttings or to the sight of blood. Nevertheless, he saw the significance in the measurements and thought of devising a method to non-invasively measure the signals from the tissues of the human body.

The same evening, while having dinner, inspiration struck Lauterbur, and he sketched his idea out on a paper napkin. He wanted to create images from the NMR signals. In order to do so, he thought of using a gradient magnetic field instead of a constant magnetic field. He thought that as the frequencies of NMR signals depended on the local magnetic field, there might be a way to locate them in a non-uniform magnetic field. He thought of creating two-dimensional pictures through this method and then stacking them to create a three-dimensional image. Paul named his technique 'zeugmatography', from the Greek word *zeugma*, meaning 'that which is used for joining'.

Even though Lauterbur and Damadian were in contact with each other, they did not collaborate to build the first MRI scanner. Sadly, a bitter rivalry ensued between the two.

Lauterbur conducted experiments on test tubes containing water and, using his gradient field approach, obtained pictures. He submitted a paper containing these images to the popular journal *Nature*, but it was rejected. He then appealed to the journal by highlighting the medical applications of the technique and its importance in the detection of cancers. His paper was subsequently accepted and published in 1973. He, however, did not cite Damadian's experiments.

Lauterbur then managed to obtain an image of a clam, which his daughter had collected during a walk at the beach. The clam was big enough to be imaged and small enough to fit in the 4 mm of available space. This was the first MRI image of a live organism. He subsequently obtained an image of the thorax of a mouse.

In order to proceed further with his experiments, he needed a human-sized magnet, for which funds were scarce. Finally, the National Cancer Institute, a part of the National Institutes of Health, provided the necessary resources. He requested a 60 cm bore magnet, but instead got a 45 cm one. The coils used to transmit and receive NMR signals had to be improved. So, the coils were made bigger, leaving only 42 cm of available space—too small to accommodate any human being.

Nevertheless, Lauterbur developed important methods and techniques to improve MRI imaging. Today, MRI machines use gradient fields along the x, y and z axes in order to obtain images in different planes.

Meanwhile, in England, physicist Peter Mansfield, working at the University of Nottingham, was using NMR gradients to study the structures of solids. After he presented a paper at a conference in Krakow in 1973, he was questioned by an editor, John Waugh, who asked if he was aware of similar work that had been published by Lauterbur a month or so earlier in the journal *Nature*. Mansfield, not a frequent reader of *Nature*, was unacquainted with Lauterbur's work. Intrigued, he searched the library for Lauterbur's paper upon his return to Nottingham. He found a huge contrast between their approaches and the fact that they were done on different materials: solids versus liquids. It then became obvious to Mansfield that it was easier to use his multiple pulse techniques on liquids rather than on solids.

He realized that point-by-point imaging would be a slow process, and this lack of speed would be a major concern for medical imaging. He thus conceived line scanning, in which a whole line of data is obtained in a one-shot experiment. This line scanning technique could be further modified to obtain an entire plane at a time. His initial setup too had limitations in size. The only living object that he could think of to fit within a diameter of 1.5 cm was a human finger. However, it turned out that his and his students' fingers were too large except for one, Andrew Maudsley. He had particularly thin fingers and the team was able to obtain images of several of his fingers. In 1976, they achieved the first human NMR scan.

On the other side of the Atlantic, Raymond Damadian set out to build his NMR machine to scan the human body. In order to build a magnet large enough to accommodate a human, he needed superconducting coils measuring around 30 miles, which would cost approximately $150,000. He only had available about $15,000. To get some technical advice, he called his friend Steve Lane at the manufacturing company Westinghouse. Lane told him that the company was exiting the business of making superconducting magnets. As a result, he had some 30 miles of superconducting wire that he could give him for $15,000—precisely the length he needed, and for the amount he had!

Within Damadian's team were Michael Goldsmith and Larry Minkoff, who had their differences. Eventually, they collaborated effectively, coming together to construct their NMR scanner and naming it 'Indomitable'.

On 24 June 1977, Damadian entered the Indomitable himself. His goal was to stay in the machine for about thirty minutes. He entered the machine with a blood pressure cuff on his arm, an EKG machine attached to his chest and a cardiologist standing by his side in case of an emergency. They tried for hours but, to their disappointment, could not receive any signal.

The next day, Goldsmith suggested that they were not receiving a signal because Damadian was 'too fat' for his coil and was loading it down. This meant that Minkoff, who was the thinnest of them all, was their best shot. Though initially reluctant—he was working on a design of his own and didn't particularly want to enter Goldsmith's coil—after observing Damadian for a while for any ill-effects that he may have had from being in the machine, Minkoff agreed and entered the machine on 2 July 1977. The team scanned for hours, finishing only at 4.45 a.m. The scan of Minkoff's torso produced 106 picture elements (pixels) in about five hours (today, an MRI generates 65,000 pixels in minutes). Minkoff was moved inch by inch while Goldsmith simultaneously drew an image on graph paper from the signal that they were receiving. The resulting image, named 'Mink 5' after Larry Minkoff, was of the heart, lungs, aorta, cardiac chamber and chest wall at the thoracic level of T8.

Around this time, Paul Lauterbur reported his setback with the inadequately sized magnet that he had received.

Meanwhile, Damadian focused on reducing the scan time and founded a company, FONAR, for the commercial production of NMR machines.

For Mansfield, his magnet arrived on the last working day before Christmas in 1977. It came in the late afternoon, during a Christmas party, and Mansfield was called to receive it. He unloaded it with two students whom he managed to drag out of the party. However, given the holiday break, they had to wait until the new year to assemble it.

After the entire machine was set up, Mansfield volunteered to be the first test subject. He climbed into the scanner and asked his teammates Peter Morris and Ian Pykett to operate it when he called out. The door of the machine was closed, and it was pitch-dark within for they hadn't installed a light inside. The wiring of the electric bulb would have interfered with the signals of the machine. As a result, Mansfield was shut inside in complete darkness with his face between two large coils that he had to make sure not to touch as they would get searing hot after a few minutes. His wife and Morris's fiancée were waiting outside, ready to pull him out in case of an emergency. Just a week before his planned scan, he had actually received a note from Professor Tom Budinger, who was a medical scientist working at the University of California, San Francisco. He had made a calculation that suggested that the gradient strength Mansfield was planning to use for his abdominal image was dangerous as it could trigger cardiac fibrillation (abnormal heart rhythm). Mansfield had done his own calculations and trusted his figures over Budinger's, so he proceeded with the scan.

Signalling his colleagues to start, Mansfield heard a loud click come from the machine, but he did not feel any discomfort. After about fifty minutes of being trapped in the sweltering heat of the machine, he got out, sweating profusely. Thankfully, the scan had gone well, resulting in the first scan of the human abdomen (since Damadian's scan was of the thorax or the chest region).

The timing was impeccable. The scan was done the night before they were due to fly out to attend the Experimental NMR Conference (ENC) meeting, which was being held in Blacksburg, Virginia, in April 1978. They took pictures of their results and carried the roll of film to the States. Once there, Mansfield got the film developed at a photo shop close to the conference centre, just in time to present his findings at the conference.

Determined to advance MRI technology further, Mansfield set up a company named General Magnetic, where, among many things, he worked on reducing the acoustic noise produced during MRIs.

Thus, it was a physicist, a chemist and a medical doctor who pioneered the field of magnetic resonance imaging. There are many more individuals who deserve credit for this magnificent discovery. The medical community remains indebted to each scientist, engineer and technician who contributed to the development of the MRI.

The Nobel Prize for Physiology or Medicine was jointly awarded to Paul Lauterbur and Peter Mansfield in the year 2003. Raymond Damadian was excluded.

As per Alfred Nobel's will, up to three individuals can share a Nobel Prize. It also stated that the physiology prize should recognize a pivotal 'discovery', while that in physics and chemistry should be given for important 'methods'. Given that Damadian discovered the differences between abnormal and normal tissues, while the other two developed imaging techniques, it remains unclear why Damadian was excluded. Some believe that the exclusion was a deliberate one due to his differences with Lauterbur and his firm belief in creation science as opposed to evolution. Unfortunately, the deliberations of the committee are kept a secret for fifty years, so we won't know the reasons that led to this decision till 2053.

After the announcement was made, Damadian, furious at his exclusion, bought full-page advertisements in *The Washington Post*, *The New York Times* and the *Los Angeles Times* to protest the decision. He also mounted a letter-writing campaign directed at Stockholm and aimed it at correcting what he called 'this shameful wrong'. Lauterbur and Mansfield, however, chose to remain silent on the issue.

There have been many other instances in the past where disputes arose over the Nobel Prize committee's decisions. For example, the decision to award Egas Moniz the Nobel Prize for prefrontal leukotomy was highly condemned.

Paul Hermann Müller was awarded the prize for his discovery of DDT, the pesticide that killed insects that spread typhus and malaria and seemed instrumental in saving millions of lives. Later, however, it was realized that DDT took a terrible toll on birds, fish and other wildlife.

Oswald T. Avery, who discovered that DNA is the chemical responsible for the transmission of inherited traits through his experiments on bacteria, was nominated for the award several times but never won.

In 1923, Frederick G. Banting and John J.R. Macleod received the prize for their discovery of insulin. Macleod, who was the department head at the University of Toronto, where the work was done, had not even been on campus when the experiments were conducted. It was Banting and a medical student, Charles Best, in collaboration with biochemist James B. Collip, who actually discovered insulin. Banting strongly acknowledged Best's contributions and shared half of his Nobel winnings with him. Inspired by Banting, Macleod split his award money with Collip.

While Damadian did not receive the Nobel Prize, his contributions were recognized elsewhere. He was awarded the nation's highest honour in technology, the United States Medal of Technology, for his invention by President Ronald Reagan. His name was also included in the National Inventors Hall of Fame, and his MRI scanner, the Indomitable, was put on display at the Smithsonian.

PET SCAN

The development of radionuclides and positron emission tomography (PET) resulted from important discoveries and advancements in physics, chemistry, physiology, mathematics and computer science, notably the discovery of computed tomography by Hounsfield. PET was the first-ever technique to allow the mapping of brain perfusion and metabolism in three dimensions. It made it possible to functionally image the brain and furthered the understanding of the various mechanisms that lead to stroke, resulting in a revolution in clinical practice.

In 1931, Paul Dirac theorized that the universe consisted not only of matter but also of antimatter as well. A year later, Caltech physicist Carl Anderson discovered the positron, the first particle of antimatter to be identified. To study cosmic rays—high-energy particles from space—he had built a cloud chamber. This instrument included a magnet, which allowed Anderson to determine whether the particles passing through were positively or negatively charged, and a lead plate to slow the particles down. He took hundreds of photographs of tracks taken by cosmic ray particles. The curve of the trajectory of one of the particles suggested that it was positively charged yet far less massive than a proton. An editor at the journal *Physical Review* suggested the name 'positron' since the particle was identical to the electron but with an opposite charge. The discovery earned Anderson the 1936 Nobel Prize in Physics. After Anderson's discovery, physicists searched through their files of cloud-chamber photographs and identified positron tracks they had previously misidentified.

The Joliot-Curies, who had earlier missed the neutron, saw that they had also missed the positron. They started up their cloud chamber again and looked for the new particle in other experimental arrangements.

The radiochemist Iréne Joliot-Curie was a battlefield radiologist, activist and politician. She also happened to be the daughter of two of the most famous scientists in the world, Marie and Pierre Curie. Jean Frédéric Joliot was a graduate of Paris's École de Physique et Chimie. In 1925, he became an assistant to Marie Curie at the Radium Institute and married Iréne in 1926. In collaboration with his wife, he performed research on the structure of the atom. They worked on the projection of the nuclei, an essential step in the discovery of the neutron and the positron. Their most important discovery was that of artificial radioactivity in 1934. They found that certain light elements emitted positrons when bombarded with alpha particles emitted from polonium. When a sheet of aluminium foil was irradiated on a polonium preparation, the emission of positrons did not cease immediately after the source was removed. The aluminium foil remained radioactive and decayed like a naturally occurring radioactive element. They observed the same phenomenon with boron and magnesium. New radioactive elements were formed by the transmutation of boron, magnesium and aluminium, named radionitrogen, radiosilicon and radiophosphorus. The couple's groundbreaking work on radioactive elements earned them the 1935 Nobel Prize in Chemistry.

Marie Curie made the following statement regarding these newly discovered radioelements: 'One could only hope that in the future one could obtain by means of tubes generating accelerated particles radioelements of which the intensity of the radiation would be comparable to that of natural radioelements.

These new substances could then have medical applications and probably other practical applications.'

In 1930, Ernest Lawrence and his colleagues in Berkeley, California, conceived the idea of a machine in which particles were accelerated between two D-shaped magnets, called a cyclotron, in order to produce progressively higher energy protons and deuterons that could then bombard elements to explore the nature of the atomic nucleus. Between 1930 and 1934, their group produced radioactive cobalt and other radionuclides by bombarding the metal components of their cyclotrons. They did not recognize the artificial radioactivity because the power supply to their cyclotron and their radiation detection instruments was shut off every evening. The report of the discovery of artificial radioactivity by the Joliot-Curies caused great disappointment within the cyclotron team because they had failed to be the first to demonstrate that one could make practically any element radioactive.

Determined to harness the capabilities of their cyclotron, the Berkeley researchers began producing artificial radionuclides in quantities that held potential for biological experiments. They produced large quantities of artificial radioisotopes, including carbon-11, nitrogen-13, oxygen-15 and fluorine-18, each of which would later prove of great significance to biomedical research. During the 1930s, biologists, physiologists and physicians flocked to Berkeley to use the newly produced radioelements as tracers. The first use of positron-emitting radionuclides in humans was done in 1945, using carbon-11-labelled carbon monoxide to study its fate in the human body.

In 1953, well before computerized tomography was invented, physicist Gordon Brownell and neurosurgeon William Sweet at Massachusetts General Hospital designed a positron scanner to localize brain tumours. This device consisted of two sodium iodide detectors mounted in columns on an adjustable platform that moved rectilinearly. A printing mechanism recorded the coincidence counting rate on carbonized paper. They used radionuclides copper-64 and arsenic-75.

In 1956, David Kuhl, a resident at the University of Pennsylvania, developed the photo scanner. In his design, a radioisotope emission-activated glow lamp provided grayscale images with greater sensitivity and resolution than ever before. Kuhl developed several single photon emission computed tomography (SPECT) devices, known as Mark II, Mark III and Mark IV, in 1964, 1970 and 1976 respectively. These early machines are considered the forerunners of SPECT, PET and CT technology.

In the mid-1950s, Michel Ter-Pogossian and his colleagues at Washington University in St. Louis worked with oxygen-15 produced by a cyclotron built in the early 1940s in the university's physics department. They studied tumours in mice. These early experiments stimulated interest in the use of short-lived radioactive gases and led, in 1955, to the building of the first medical cyclotron located on the grounds of Hammersmith Hospital in London. This was followed by installations at Massachusetts General Hospital and Washington University's Mallinckrodt Institute of Radiology in 1965. Subsequently, the US Department of Energy funded hospital cyclotrons at UCLA, the University of Chicago and Memorial Sloan Kettering Cancer Center in New York. Existing cyclotrons at UC Berkeley and Ohio State continued to be used to produce radionuclides of biological importance. Worldwide, medical cyclotrons were soon installed at McGill University in Montreal, Canada, and at the Frédéric Joliot Clinical Research Hospital in Orsay, France. Inspired by the introduction of the X-ray CT scan by Hounsfield in 1972, Ter-Pogossian and his team realized that if an image of the density of a transverse section of the body could be reconstructed from the measured attenuation of highly focused X-ray beams projected through the section, as in a CT scanner, then the distribution of a radionuclide within the section could also be accurately and quantitatively reconstructed from its emissions. This resulted in the design and construction of a machine for positron emission tomography, christened positron emission transaxial tomography (PETT). The term 'transaxial' was later dropped. The prototypical PETT I and PETT II were table-top models. They were then expanded to the clinically applicable PETT III whole body camera. Eventually the PETT V and PETT VI were developed. The PET VI was commissioned in 1980 and was developed strictly for the brain. It could handle very high-count rates and gave quick measurements. The majority of techniques for brain mapping were developed on the PETT VI. It was decommissioned as a human instrument in 1993 but is still used for animal studies. In parallel, Michael Phelps at UCLA developed the ECAT PET scanner with an industrial partner, and the first-ever commercial ECAT scanner. It was delivered to Orsay, France, in late 1977 and was routinely used in human studies in early 1978.

During the late 1980s and onwards, the advent of diffusion/perfusion MRI and advanced CT techniques replaced PET as a clinical tool for evaluating stroke patients. Brain PET has largely remained a research tool for analysing brain function and metabolism, currently by means of PET/MR hybrid scanners.

9

Thunderclap

When the thunderclap comes, there is no time to cover the ears.

—Sun Tzu

It's called the silent killer because it's often very difficult to know that you have an aneurysm. Your first symptom is often your last.

—Jeffery Carpenter

I had just finished filming Season 1 of Game of Thrones. Then I was struck with the first of two aneurysms.

—Emilia Clarke

THE BRAIN IS enveloped by three membranes, or meninges, inside the skull. The outermost of these is the dura mater (tough mother), which is closest to the skull. Below this is the arachnoid mater, named so because of its spider web-like appearance. The innermost layer is the pia mater (tender mother), a delicate membrane that adheres tightly to the brain, following all its contours. In between the arachnoid and the pia mater is the subarachnoid space, which extends continuously down to the spinal cord and contains the cerebrospinal fluid. This fluid provides a cushioning effect to the brain. However, complications can arise when there is bleeding into the subarachnoid space, following trauma or just spontaneously. The most common cause of spontaneous bleeding is the rupturing of an aneurysm (aneurysmal dilatation).

To visualize an aneurysm, picture a garden hosepipe. If you were to cut a hole in it and attach a balloon to that opening, the balloon would eventually fill with water. If the pressure of the water were too high, the balloon would burst. The pipe is your blood vessel and the balloon an aneurysm. The aneurysm may be projecting out of the vessel with a stalk or could be present circumferentially. The former is a saccular or berry aneurysm and the latter a fusiform one. This abnormal dilatation may be present since birth or can develop over time.

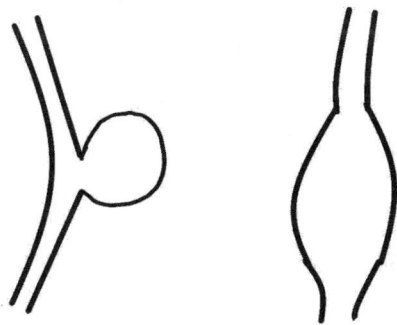

Saccular Aneurysm   *Fusiform Aneurysm*

Figure 6 The two types of aneurysms

The rupturing of these aneurysms in the subarachnoid space leads to subarachnoid haemorrhage (SAH). The primary symptom is a sudden, intense headache, known as a thunderclap headache, which is often described by patients as the worst headache of their lives. This headache may or may not be associated with loss of consciousness, nausea or vomiting. Around 10 to 15 per cent of individuals affected by this condition die before even reaching a hospital.

The rigid nature of the skull offers little room for the brain to expand. As blood from the ruptured aneurysm collects, it clots and exerts pressure on the brain, crushing it against the skull or causing it to herniate. The by-products formed as the blood breaks down irritate the wall of the blood vessel and cause it to go into a state of spasm (known as vosospasm), and it becomes very narrow. The part of the brain away from the site of rupture that was to be supplied oxygen-rich blood by the rupturing artery will be deprived of blood. This could lead to a secondary stroke. Thus, medical treatment is aimed at alleviating the symptoms of headache, preventing seizures, preventing vasospasm and decreasing the pressure on the brain. A ruptured aneurysm is very likely to bleed again, hence the definitive treatment is to treat the aneurysm.

Game of Thrones' star Emilia Clarke had to deal with complications associated with brain aneurysms in 2011 and then in 2013. She hid her story from her fans for eight years, until she finally decided to make it public in an interview with *The New Yorker* in 2019. 'Just when all my childhood dreams seemed to have come true, I nearly lost my mind and then my life. I've never told this story publicly, but now it's time.'

On 11 February 2011, while working out, Clarke felt the onset of a headache and took a break, going to the locker room. As she recalled:

> I reached the toilet, sank to my knees, and proceeded to be violently, voluminously ill. Meanwhile, the pain—shooting, stabbing, constricting pain—was getting worse. At some level, I knew what was happening: my brain was damaged ... I heard a woman's voice coming from the next stall, asking me if I was O.K. No, I wasn't. She came to help me and maneuvered me onto my side, in the recovery position. Then everything became, at once, noisy and blurry. I remember the sound of a siren, an ambulance; I heard new voices, someone saying that my pulse was weak.

She was taken to the emergency room of Whittington Hospital, where an MRI revealed a subarachnoid haemorrhage due to an aneurysm rupture. She needed emergency repair of the aneurysm.

> I remember being told that I should sign a release form for surgery. Brain surgery? I was in the middle of my very busy life—I had no *time* for brain surgery. But, finally, I settled down and signed. And then I was unconscious. For the next three hours, surgeons went about repairing my brain. This would not be my last surgery and it would not be the worst. I was twenty-four years old.

Clarke recalled having suffered from a migraine at the age of fourteen, one that kept her in bed for a couple of days, and that she'd collapse in drama school once in a while. These could have been the warning signs of her aneurysm.

The first surgery that Clarke underwent was minimally invasive—the surgeons did not open her skull. It was an endovascular approach, which happens through the vessels. The surgeons passed catheters through the femoral artery in her groin, to her heart and from there, progressed them to the arteries in the brain till they reached the aneurysm. They repaired the aneurysm by coiling it with a wire.

> 'The operation lasted three hours. When I woke, the pain was unbearable. I had no idea where I was. My field of vision was constricted. There was a tube down my throat and I was parched and nauseated. They moved me out of the I.C.U. after four days and told me that the great hurdle was to make it to the two-week mark. If I made it that long with minimal complications, my chances of a good recovery were high. One night after I'd passed that crucial mark, a nurse woke me and, as part of a series of cognitive exercises, she said, 'What's your name?' My full name is Emilia Isobel Euphemia Rose Clarke. But now I couldn't remember it. Instead, nonsense words tumbled out of my mouth, and I went into a blind panic. I'd never experienced fear like that—a sense of doom closing in. I could see my life ahead, and it wasn't worth living. I am an actor; I need to remember my lines. Now I couldn't recall my name.'

Clarke was suffering from aphasia due to brain damage. She was sent back to the ICU. Fortunately, about a week later, her aphasia passed and she could speak again. She stayed in the hospital for about a month. 'I left the hospital, longing for a bath and fresh air. I had press interviews to do and in a matter of weeks, I was scheduled to be back on the set of *Game of Thrones*.'

Clarke had another aneurysm on the other side of her brain, which was at risk of 'popping' at any moment. However, it was small, and there was a possibility that it would indefinitely remain dormant and harmless. But she needed to undergo regular brain scans to keep a watch on the aneurysm.

In 2013, Clarke underwent the brain scan. Unfortunately, the aneurysm on the other side of the brain had doubled in size and her doctors said that they 'should take care of it'. She was to undergo another minimally invasive operation. But the operation failed, and she had a massive bleed in the brain, for which the doctors had to open her skull.

> I emerged from the operation with a drain coming out of my head. Bits of my skull had been replaced by titanium. These days, you can't see the scar that curves from my scalp to my ear, but I didn't know at first that it wouldn't be visible. And there was, above all, the constant worry about cognitive or sensory losses. Would it be concentration? Memory? Peripheral vision? Now I tell people that what it robbed me of is good taste in men. But, of course, none of this was remotely funny at the time.

Clarke was discharged about six weeks after the surgery. She not only made her story public but also founded a charity, SameYou, to fund treatment for people recovering from brain injuries and stroke.

Historically, tying the carotid artery in the neck on the side of the brain aneurysm was the primary treatment for cerebral aneurysms. However, the results were often variable and unpredictable. Astley Cooper (1786–1841) reported two cases of carotid artery aneurysms, which he treated with ligation. The first patient, who had a massive carotid aneurysm occupying two-thirds of her neck, developed hemiplegia soon after the operation and died shortly thereafter. In contrast, the second patient, with a considerably smaller aneurysm, was treated successfully and returned to employment eight months after the surgery. In 1885, Victor Horsley (1857–1916), while operating on a patient with a suspected brain tumour, accidentally discovered a massive aneurysm in the middle cranial fossa. He successfully ligated the cervical carotid artery, and the patient was reported to be in good health even five years after.

Harvey Cushing (1869–1939) is heralded as the father of modern neurological surgery, and his portrait brands the American Association of Neurological Surgeons. Born into a long line of physicians, including his father, grandfather and great-grandfather, Cushing obtained his undergraduate degree from Yale Medical School in 1891 and completed his medical training at Harvard, graduating in 1895. He then studied under William Stewart Halsted at Johns Hopkins until 1912. From there, he moved to Harvard as the chief of surgery at the Peter Bent Brigham Hospital.

As a medical student in 1895, Cushing, along with a classmate, Ernest Amory Codman, developed the forerunner of the modern anaesthetic record used today to monitor temperature, heart rate and blood pressure during surgery. In an illustrious career, Cushing would author more than 300 articles and thirteen books. His major interest was brain tumours, and between 1912 and 1938, he published five books on his study and treatment of 2,023 confirmed tumours. In the history of the development of neuro-oncology, no individual has surpassed the contributions of Cushing. They include an understanding of the dynamics of intracranial pressure (ICP), the development of the pathological classification of glioma and, at the age of sixty-three, the description of pituitary basophilia (Cushing syndrome). His contributions to other fields were also numerous. In 1926, he was awarded the Pulitzer Prize for his book, *The Life of Sir William Osler*. Additionally, his work *A Bio-Bibliography of Andreas Vesalius* remains a definitive work in this field.

Cushing, in the 'little black book' (a register which recorded the outcomes of his surgical procedures), documented the operative details and clinical outcomes of nine patients with suspected brain tumours, who were found to harbour cerebral aneurysms during his exploratory craniotomies. He would puncture the pulsating mass with a lumbar needle and the gush of blood would confirm the diagnosis of an aneurysm. He would then wrap the aneurysm with strands of muscle to control the bleeding and promote clot formation. However, he did not consider carotid ligation safe and reliable, and would rarely and very reluctantly perform it due to a high number of patients developing hemiparesis because of the abrupt stoppage of blood supply to the brain.

In a bid to control complications associated with carotid ligation, gradual carotid occlusion was attempted. The idea was to promote thrombosis within the aneurysmal sac while allowing the development of collateral circulation (other arteries taking over the function of that carotid artery). This was achieved with a Selverstone clamp, a stainless-steel clamp that could be placed around the carotid artery and tightened to occlude the vessel. Tools that were fastened to the clamp and passed through the tissues to the surface of the skin were used to tighten the clamp or to open it, should the patient show any signs of insufficient collateral circulation. The artery was to be occluded over a period of seventy-two hours and the clamp was given a quarter turn a day. While it had fewer ischemic complications compared to traditional carotid ligation, the overall results were less than encouraging.

Norman Dott (1897–1973), one of Cushing's residents, was the first to successfully treat a ruptured internal carotid aneurysm by wrapping it with a muscle. He then went ahead and perfected a highly technical and hazardous technique of ligating the neck of the aneurysm with a suture. Sutures were notoriously difficult to secure and could easily rupture the friable aneurysm wall. Cushing, in 1911, designed a silver clip to control deep and inaccessible blood vessels during brain tumour resection. Despite designing it, he never actually used it to secure cerebral aneurysms. This clip was modified, and the first successful clipping was performed by his competitor Walter Dandy in 1937. This marked the birth of modern vascular neurosurgery, the basic principles of which form the backbone of cerebral aneurysm surgery practised today.

However, due to suboptimal instruments, a lack of magnification and primitive neuro-anaesthesia, many surgeons continued to advise bed rest or practise carotid ligation up until the 1970s. Subsequently, with the development of the operative microscope and improvements in the designs of the clips, many areas of the brain previously considered inaccessible became approachable. Subsequent studies demonstrated significantly reduced death rates with aneurysm surgery as compared to conservative management and carotid ligation.

In 1864, Charles Moore and Charles Murchison, inspired by the clinical observation of a fibrin-coated bullet recovered during an autopsy, postulated that inserting a wire into an aneurysm would provide an ideal environment for clot production, which would occlude the aneurysm. Thus, if a large quantity of wire could be introduced into the interior of an aneurysm and disposed about in coils, a corresponding amount of fibrin would soon accumulate and increase upon it. Progressively, the fibrin would adhere tightly to the vessel wall and seal the aneurysm. The wire would remain in the aneurysm, enveloped in the clot, but be harmless.

To test their theory, Moore and Murchison focused on a thoracic aortic aneurysm, evident as a large, pulsating mass in the chest. They introduced twenty-six yards of a very fine iron wire into the aneurysm, which resulted in clinical improvement, a reduction in the size of the aneurysm and a decrease in the pulse rate from 116 to 92 beats per minute. Though the patient eventually died of infection, at the autopsy, the coils of wire were found filled with 'fibrinous coagulum' and were 'firmly adherent'. The idea found widespread application but had certain short- and long-term complications, like risk of haemorrhage from subtotal packing and distal embolization of wire or thrombus. Moreover, it was a percutaneous (through the skin) approach. This meant that surgery could only be performed in an aneurysm that could be easily reached through the surface of the body and not those in deeper arteries. It was effective for saccular aneurysms but not fusiform ones.

Electrothrombosis, or galvanopuncture, was a technique that introduced electric currents to induce thrombosis. The mechanisms suggested included inflammation, oxidation or albumin decomposition following the passage of the current. In 1879, Alfonso Corradi tried combining wire insertion and electrothrombosis. However, the mortality rates following the procedure were high, and it was subsequently abandoned.

Concurrent advances in neurosurgery allowed for a combined approach, through which the aneurysm was surgically exposed and a wire was inserted through a trocar.

Although these initial attempts made by these pioneers yielded limited success—mainly because the tools used to navigate the complex intracranial vasculature were lacking—they laid the foundation for current endovascular treatment for intracranial aneurysms. The desire for an alternative to conventional surgery and technological advancements facilitated a shift from an extravascular to an endovascular approach. In order to use blood vessels as natural conduits into the vascular lesions of the brain, various delivery systems, or microcatheters, were developed. The major obstacles in the safe catheterization of brain arteries were the tortuosity, narrowness and delicacy of the intracranial arteries.

In 1964, a breakthrough occurred when two neurosurgeons from Georgetown University Hospital in Washington, DC, Luessenhop and Velasquez, documented the first catheterization of a brain vessel. They used a glass chamber, surgically connected to the external carotid artery, to deliver a length of silastic tubing into the internal carotid artery and thereby into the brain arteries. In one patient, the distal tip of the catheter was inflated like a balloon to temporarily block the neck of a large posterior communicating artery aneurysm. They stated that 'intraluminal manipulation of the intracranial arteries about the circle of Willis is possible technically and is tolerated by these arteries'.

Later, in 1966, Frei et al. designed a para-operational device catheter for super selective catheterization with minimum vessel trauma. The catheter tip had an attached micromagnet. External magnetic fields could be applied to direct the micromagnet-tipped catheter through the tortuous intracranial vessels. A continuous magnetic field would pull it while an alternating field would cause it to vibrate. The net effect was to induce the catheter to 'swim' within the vessels by reducing the friction between the catheter tip and the inner vessel wall.

A significant invention that revolutionized the endovascular treatment of intracranial aneurysms was the detachable balloon. In 1974, Fedor A. Serbinenko published the results of 300 patients with arteriovenous malformations and cerebral aneurysms treated with microcatheter balloons. This work had an exceptional influence on endovascular neurosurgeons, who conducted their own experiments with various modifications. The problem with the balloon system, however, was that the balloons were mostly spherical, while aneurysms came in various shapes. Balloons filled with rigid materials forced the aneurysms to adapt to their shape. Although the outcomes using the balloon-based approach were markedly improved as compared to previous methods, there was a high incidence of immediate complications, including delayed rupture of the aneurysm and recanalization.

The substantial failure of balloon embolization prompted investigators to find a less traumatic embolic agent that could gently adopt the shape of the aneurysm. The use of short pushable coils for endosaccular packing was reported by Hilal in 1988. However, these coils were relatively stiff, and a dense packing of the aneurysm could not be achieved. Furthermore, as these coils were non-retrievable, the probability of deposition in the parent artery was high.

Guido Guglielmi, during his experiments on electrothrombosis, noticed that a stainless-steel wire would get eroded when a current was passed, a phenomenon known as electrolysis. By attaching an electrolysis-resistant platinum coil to the stainless-steel wire, Guglielmi invented the concept of the detachable coil, going on to successfully treat his first patient in 1990. Numerous coils can be deposited in the aneurysm using this method. The aneurysm is slowly and gently filled with coils until it is completely and tightly packed. The detachable coils adapt to the shape of the aneurysm and are less deforming than a balloon.

With the emergence of the technique of coiling, there arose an intense debate between the advocates of coiling and those in favour of clipping, which prompted the International Subarachnoid Aneurysm Trial. The results of the trial showed that coiling was associated with less mortality and morbidity than clipping. The various advancements in the techniques of coiling made over the past few years include the development of balloon-assisted coiling, stent-assisted coiling and flow diverters.

10

'Time Is Brain'

> *The old wives' tale was that you had one stroke, and then you sat around waiting for a second one, or a third one, or however many it took to kill you. If you had any kind of brain injury affecting your locomotive functions, everyone assumed your life was finished.*
>
> —Howard A. Rusk

ON 25 JULY 1989, President George Bush, in response to reports from the National Advisory Councils of the National Institute of Neurological Disorders and Stroke (NINDS) and the National Institute of Mental Health (NIMH), and at the urging of Congress, signed a presidential declaration designating the 1990s to be the 'Decade of the Brain', calling on the United States to observe the decade with appropriate activities. The goal was to 'enhance public awareness of the benefits to be derived from brain research'. This declaration led to international communities adopting the movement as well. The government of Japan invested $125 million into neuroscience research in

1997, leading to the development of the Brain Science Institute. The government of India founded the National Brain Research Centre in the same year. In 1998, the Chinese Institute of Neuroscience was founded.

The Decade of the Brain witnessed a change of attitude among neurologists in the treatment of stroke. A stroke is now treated as a medical emergency, just like a heart attack or head trauma. Before the availability of imaging techniques like CT scans and MRI, or clot-dissolving drugs and interventional techniques to remove clots, there was limited recourse for a stroke patient.

I would emphasise again here that it has been estimated that a patient loses 1.9 million neurons each minute if the brain is deprived of its blood supply, and thus 'time is brain'.

Imagine a garden equipped with regularly spaced water sprinklers. There will be some amount of overlap between the areas supplied by two sprinklers. If one of the sprinklers breaks down, the grass that is exclusively fed by it and just around it would dry up the fastest, while the grass slightly farther away from that sprinkler will receive a little water from the surrounding sprinklers and could still survive. Similarly, when an artery is blocked, as in an ischemic stroke, survival of the at-risk tissue depends upon the duration and intensity of the ischemia and the availability of collateral blood flow from other nearby arteries. The degree of ischemia caused by the blockage of an artery varies in different zones supplied by that artery. In the centre of the zone, blood flow is the lowest, and the ischemic damage is most severe. This region of the most severe damage is often referred to as the 'core' of the infarct. On the periphery of the affected area, collateral blood flow allows some delivery of blood. This peripheral zone becomes dysfunctional, but it is not dead and has traditionally been referred to as the ischemic penumbra. Swift restoration of blood supply can potentially save the neurons in the penumbra.

Therapy with clot-dissolving drugs like rtPA is only effective if given within three to four and a half hours following stroke onset. The availability of interventional techniques to mechanically remove clots can extend this therapeutic window a little longer, up to twenty-four hours. Since the benefits of rtPA are time dependent, various guidelines recommend a door-to-needle time of sixty minutes or less. Thus, when a patient arrives at the emergency room, doctors rush to stabilize them and obtain a CT scan to determine if the stroke is ischemic or haemorrhagic. A haemorrhagic stroke is easily visible on a CT scan and its treatment is entirely different from that of an ischemic stroke. A patient can't be given rtPA unless a haemorrhage is ruled out on a CT scan, as it can increase bleeding. If there is no haemorrhage and the stroke is ischemic, clot-dissolving drugs are administered immediately, as long as the patient has no contraindications to its use.

If the stroke is haemorrhagic, the goal of the treatment is to stop the bleeding in the hours immediately after the haemorrhage. The accumulated blood can cause pressure on the surrounding structures and can also lead to swelling around the brain. Since hypertension is the most common cause of bleeding in the brain, it is important to reduce high blood pressure in these patients. In some patients, the bleeding is due to an excess of blood thinners. There are many drugs available that can reverse the effects of blood thinners. In some patients, the bleeding might be excessive, and they may need to undergo surgical treatment to remove the blood accumulated in the brain.

BLS/ACLS

Medical students, interns, doctors and nurses are required to undergo training and be certified to provide basic life support (BLS) and advanced cardiac life support (ACLS). These courses, designed by the American Heart Association (AHA), mandate recertification every two years. I've completed this training thrice so far. It is the same standard course in India and the United States.

BLS training equips individuals to promptly recognize life-threatening conditions, such as a heart attack, and give the victim the best chance of survival till medical help is obtained. Its main principles are giving high-quality chest compressions, delivering appropriate ventilations and providing the early use of an automated external defibrillator (AED). When someone's heart suddenly stops, the blood supply to vital organs, such as the brain, is compromised. A BLS provider's chest compressions temporarily take over the heart's role in pumping blood to vital organs. Artificial breaths are given in between these chest compressions to maintain the oxygenation of the blood. In cases where heart failure is due to abnormal rhythms of the heart, such as ventricular fibrillation and pulseless ventricular tachycardia, an AED can be used—they are usually available at public sites. An AED recognizes these abnormal rhythms and delivers a shock that stops the abnormal rhythm and allows the heart to re-establish an effective rhythm.

The AHA stands as the oldest and biggest voluntary health organization in the United States committed to combatting cardiovascular diseases and stroke. Its story began back in 1915, when a team of pioneers made up of social workers and physicians established the first association for the prevention and relief of heart disease in New York City. A lack of knowledge about heart disease made it difficult for patients to go on with their lives, and they were often put on bed rest. After conducting various studies to determine if patients could go back to work, these physicians inspired colleagues across the nation and Canada to form other heart associations in the 1920s. The increased interest in heart disease and a number of similar organizations emphasized the need for one national organization that would encourage further research. With that goal, six cardiologists, all members of different groups, joined their efforts in 1924. This is how the AHA was founded.

As a provider of valuable information about stroke and heart disease, the AHA's goal was to effectively prevent and treat cardiovascular diseases, ultimately saving lives and building healthier communities. With the help of dedicated scientists, physicians and healthcare providers worldwide, the AHA has formed proven strategies and programmes for emergency cardiovascular care.

Half a century after the organization was formed, and after several landmark studies, the AHA recognized the need to transfer its findings from clinics and laboratories to doctors' offices and eventually to households. In 1974, the AHA published its first guidelines for ACLS certification.

While BLS can be taught to anyone, ACLS requires extensive training and practise and can only be performed by qualified and certified healthcare professionals.

ACLS builds on the foundation of BLS and consists of a series of protocols used to treat life-threatening emergencies. These interventions have been forged from expert consensus, extensive research and clinical and case studies. It equips students with the skills required to recognize and intervene in cases of heart failure, stroke, abnormal heart rhythms and respiratory arrest. This takes place through both theoretical instruction and simulation exercises.

ACT FAST!

'FAST' is a mnemonic designed to help detect and enhance responsiveness to the needs of a person having a stroke. It stands for:

F: Facial drooping—a section of the face, usually on one side, that droops and becomes hard to move. This can be recognized by a crooked smile.

A: Arm weakness—an inability to raise one's arm fully, or an inability to hold something or squeeze something, such as someone's hand.

S: Speech difficulties—an inability or difficulty to understand or produce speech, slurred speech or difficulty repeating even a basic sentence, such as 'The sky is blue.'

T: Time to call emergency services. If any of the above symptoms show up in an individual, it is essential to call emergency services and go to the hospital immediately. It is also important to check the time, so that the moment of onset and the duration of the symptoms are known before administrating rtPA.

FAST was developed in the UK in 1998 by a group of stroke physicians, ambulance personnel and an emergency department physician, and was designed to be an integral part of a training package for ambulance staff. The mnemonic was created to expedite the administration of intravenous rtPA to patients within three hours of acute stroke symptom onset.

A modification of FAST is BE-FAST, which looks at two additional symptoms:

B: Balance—sudden loss of balance or coordination

E: Eyes—sudden blurred, double or loss of vision

Stroke Units and Stroke Centres

During the nineteenth and the first two-thirds of the twentieth century, nearly all acute stroke patients were cared for in the general wards and rooms of hospitals. During the 1960s and '70s, neurology departments began to split off from departments of internal medicine within academic centres in the United States and Europe. When this occurred, hospitals with neurology departments began to place stroke patients in neurology wards and private rooms.

In the 1980s and '90s, specialized stroke units took root. These units were composed of nurses with training in stroke, internists and stroke neurologists. The care provided in these units was multifaceted: specialized nursing care, rigorous blood pressure management, protocols to facilitate rapid and thorough evaluation and treatment, monitored treatment, randomized therapeutic trials, and education on stroke and its prevention for patients and their families and caregivers. They also promoted an up-beat, optimistic view of stroke recovery, in contrast to the situation previously present in medical wards, where stroke patients were often considered unlikely to recover. Dedicated stroke units decreased mortality, limited stroke morbidity and allowed more patients to retain their independence and return home after a stroke.

The evolution of stroke care took another step when the Brain Attack Coalition (BAC) was formed in 1996. As a multidisciplinary organization, BAC brought together most major medical organizations involved with stroke care in the United States. BAC members determined that two levels of stroke centres should be established: a primary stroke centre (PSC) and a comprehensive stroke centre (CSC).

A PSC's role is to stabilize and provide emergency care for patients with acute stroke. The major elements of a PSC are acute stroke teams, written protocols, emergency medical services, stroke units, neurological services and imaging techniques. These centres would then either transfer the patient to a CSC or would admit the patient and provide further care, depending on the patient's need and that centre's capabilities.

On the other hand, a CSC would include tertiary care medical centres and hospitals furnished with the infrastructure and personnel necessary to perform highly technical procedures like thrombectomies and provide all needed levels of care. Studies have affirmed the benefits of PSCs and CSCs in improving outcomes for admitted patients. The joint commission and other national, regional and state agencies have developed and implemented certification programmes for PSCs and CSCs.

In 2013, BAC proposed a new designation for hospitals that are not yet PSCs but can provide timely, evidence-based care to most patients suffering an acute stroke: the Acute Stroke Ready Hospital (ASRH). The ASRH would provide initial diagnostic services, stabilization and emergency care and then transfer the patients to a PSC or CSC. An ASRH would not require a stroke unit of its own.

Mobile Stroke Unit (MSU)

The concept of a mobile stroke unit (MSU) was first published by Fassbender et al. in 2003 as a way of 'bringing treatment to the patient rather than the patient to the treatment'. All MSUs have the basic components to provide assessment and treatment of acute ischemic infarcts, including standard ambulance equipment and medications, a computed tomography (CT) scanner, point-of-care laboratory equipment, telemedicine capabilities and tPA. In addition to the staff of a standard ambulance, the unit also has a physician, either in person or through telemedicine, and a member trained as a CT technologist. In the first generation of MSUs, standard ambulances could not house all the necessary components, but miniaturization of technology has now allowed everything to fit into a standard ambulance. The team members work to quickly and effectively diagnose or rule out stroke and determine tPA eligibility. It eliminates the delays associated with in-hospital care, such as triage of multiple patients, competing obligations of the hospitalist, availability of a CT scanner and the divided attention of emergency department nurses and technicians.

11

Abilities versus Disabilities

The brain is a far more open system than we ever imagined, and nature has gone very far to help us perceive and take in the world around us. It has given us a brain that survives in a changing world by changing itself.

—Norman Doidge

The human brain, it has been said, is the most complexly organised structure in the universe and to appreciate this you just have to look at some numbers. The brain is made up of one hundred billion nerve cells or 'neurons' which are the basic structural and functional units of the nervous system. Each neuron makes something like a thousand to ten thousand contacts with other neurons and these points of contact are called synapses where exchange of information occurs. And based on this information, someone has calculated that the number of possible permutations and combinations of brain activity, in other words the number of brain states, exceeds the number of elementary particles in the known universe.

— V.S. Ramachandran

PHYSICAL MEDICINE AND rehabilitation (PM&R) emerged as a speciality in the first half of the twentieth century, with significant growth and development stimulated by the World Wars and severe epidemics of paralytic poliomyelitis. Physicians and therapists were needed to treat the soldiers returning from war with serious injuries and chronic disabling conditions. The availability of antibiotics and improved surgical techniques during World War II allowed more injured soldiers to survive, albeit with significant disabilities. Amongst civilians, severe epidemics of polio combined with industrial and motor vehicle accidents were a major cause of disability. These events necessitated the development of new restorative treatment programmes incorporating new physical and rehabilitative techniques, and the establishment of training programmes for physicians and therapists to administer these treatments.

Franklin Delano Roosevelt (1882–1945), the most famous victim of polio, played an important role in the development of rehabilitation medicine. He contracted the disease in the summer of 1921 and was left paralysed from the waist down. Despite his disability, he pursued his political aspirations and, in 1932, was elected president of the United States. Roosevelt's journey not only helped eradicate some of the social stigma associated with physical disability, but also provided inspiration and hope, promoting the idea that polio victims could be 'normal' again. His leadership catalysed social action and philanthropy for those with disabilities. In 1927, Roosevelt founded the Georgia Warm Springs Foundation, which helped develop physical therapy and rehabilitation approaches for polio victims. In 1937, the foundation was reorganized as the National Foundation for Infantile Paralysis under the direction of Roosevelt's former law partner, Basil O'Connor. This foundation held a highly successful fundraising campaign utilizing an annual 'President's Birthday Ball'. The campaign was labelled 'March of Dimes' and generated extraordinary interest, raising an unprecedented $268,000 in 1938. Through the patronage of the National Foundation, an extensive nationwide biomedical initiative was orchestrated. This initiative subsidized the hospital and rehabilitation costs of polio patients, funded basic and applied research concerning the causes and prevention of polio in the 1940s and early '50s, trained nurses and physical therapists in rehabilitation, sponsored pilot programmes to improve the teaching of rehabilitation medicine in medical schools and, ultimately, underwrote the Salk Vaccine Field Trial in 1954.

In the late nineteenth and early twentieth centuries, most medical investigations concerning stroke were focused on its pathology and clinical presentation. At this time, very little effort was dedicated to the rehabilitation of stroke victims. Initial approaches were rudimentary. For people with speech loss, rehabilitation consisted of repetitive reading, spelling and word repetition exercises. For those with varying degrees of physical paralysis, passive movements or light exercise programmes were conducted. Various orthotic and assistive devices, such as splints to prevent contractures, light braces for support, canes, crutches and wheelchairs, were used.

Rehabilitation for stroke victims was not systematically developed until the second half of the twentieth century. In the 1970s and '80s, the stroke rehabilitation team approach began to develop and spread. Stroke units were assembled in larger hospitals and urban areas, facilitating a seamless transition between acute care and rehabilitation. Outpatient rehabilitation resources were developed, including services provided by health departments, visiting nurse associations, day care centres, and hospital-associated and independent physical therapy practices.

NEUROPLASTICITY

For most of the twentieth century, the structure of the brain and spinal cord in adults was believed to be hard-wired and unchanging, no matter what rehabilitation or environmental influence was applied after damage. This traditional view was overturned by the experiments of Edward Taub. As Taub worked towards transforming stroke rehabilitation at his lab in Silver Spring, Maryland, he was unaware that his test animals would become the most famous in the history of research.

Edward Taub was born in 1931 in Brooklyn. He studied behaviourism under Fred Keller at Columbia University before going on to take a job as a research assistant in a neurology lab, where he got involved in deafferentation experiments with primates. Our nervous system has a sensory component and a motor component. The sensory component comprises nerves that carry impulses from the sensory organs, such as the skin, eyes and ears, to the brain and the spinal cord. These are the afferent (towards the centre) nerves. Deafferentation is a procedure in which the spinal cord is opened surgically and these sensory or afferent nerves are severed.

Taub, with the help of a neurosurgeon, deafferented one side of some monkeys' limbs, keeping the other side intact. Post-procedure, the monkeys were unable to perceive any sensations of pain, touch or temperature in those limbs and began treating them as if they were detached from their bodies and were foreign objects. Since the monkeys did not feel any pain, they ended up injuring their arms and even tried biting them. The monkeys used only their good arms for feeding or other purposes. Taub described it as the 'learned non-use' of the deafferented arm, for it was a learning phenomenon involving conditioned suppression of movement.

The deafferentation procedure involved the severing of only the sensory nerves, but after the procedure both the sensory and motor neurons in the spinal cord were unable to fire for about two to six months. This was due to the spinal cord going into a state of shock. Recovery from spinal shock required considerable time, and the use of the affected extremity during this time led to incoordination and accidents, such as dropping of food items and general failure of any activity attempted by the monkeys. The animals gradually learnt to balance on three limbs and used the intact limb for eating. Thus, punishment associated with the use of the deafferented limbs and positive enforcement with the use of the unaffected limbs led to the learned non-use of the deafferented limb. And even though the motor function returned in the deafferented limb after a few months, the monkeys failed to recognize that the limb was potentially useful again.

Taub conducted a series of these deafferentation experiments. In one study, he constrained the use of the unaffected limb by applying a sling to it, so the monkey was forced to use the deafferented limb to reach out for food in order to survive. In another experiment, he deafferented both the limbs of a monkey, but, to his surprise, the monkey was able to use both. In yet another experiment, instead of constraining the good limb, Taub constrained the deafferented limb during the spinal shock phase.

When he removed the sling three months later, the monkey was able to use the limb after some time. Taub concluded that by eliminating both punishment and reward, the function of the deafferented limb returned. He then applied this concept of learned non-use to stroke patients and developed constraint-induced movement therapy (CIMT) as a method to counteract this behaviour.

While undergoing CIMT therapy, the good, or working hand of a patient is restricted with the help of a mitt or a sling and the patient is asked to perform various activities with the side affected by stroke. It starts with small attempts at movements of the fingers and is gradually progressed to more complex movements, such as reaching to grasp a cup of coffee. The repeated practice and restriction of the good side stimulate the brain to overcome learned non-use and to reorganize itself.

The reason Taub's Silver Spring monkeys earned fame was not because of his research but because their treatment by Taub and his team came under fire from People for the Ethical Treatment of Animals, or PETA.

In May 1981, Taub was approached by Alex Pacheco, a graduate student at George Washington University, who asked if he could volunteer at Taub's lab. Pacheco, the son of a doctor, was raised in Mexico and initially wanted to become a priest. He underwent a major transformation after visiting a slaughterhouse and reading Peter Singer's *Animal Liberation*. He stopped eating meat and collaborated with Ingrid Newkirk, a local pound master, to form PETA in 1980. In order to gain firsthand insights into animal research labs, he decided to work in one. He chose Taub's lab as it was closest to his home and government funded. Taub offered him an unpaid position at his lab. As Norman Doidge wrote, 'When Pacheco volunteered to work with Taub, his goal was to free the seventeen Silver Spring Monkeys and make them a rallying cry for an animal rights campaign.'

In the summer of 1981, when Taub was away on a three-week vacation, Pacheco photographed the lab, documenting the animals' filthy living conditions. He alleged that the monkey cages had not been cleaned in a long time and that they were filled with faeces and urine. He said that the monkeys were underfed and were picking scraps of food from the waste tray placed below the cages. Since the monkeys could not feel their limbs, they were severely injured. Most of the injuries were self-inflicted, as the animals tried to bite their arms, now foreign to them. According to Pacheco, no one bothered to bandage the limbs or apply antibiotics to the monkeys' wounds. Leveraging these allegations against Taub, he persuaded Maryland authorities and the local police to raid the lab and seize the monkeys. The raid received extensive media coverage and presented Taub as cruel and barbaric.

When Taub returned, he was horrified by what had transpired in his absence. He was arrested and charged with 119 counts of animal cruelty and failure to provide veterinary care. The National Institutes of Health (NIH), fearful of being PETA's next target, turned against Taub and suspended his $115,000 research grant. The repercussions for Taub were profound and extended into his personal life, with death threats to him and his wife.

In his defence, Taub argued that he had been framed. He insisted that his lab had been clean when he left for vacation and that Pacheco himself had failed to clean the cages or care for the animals in Taub's absence, and then presented false reports. Taub pointed out that during his vacation, two of his employees who were supposed to clean the lab and feed the animals were absent for a week—this was unusual given their consistent attendance over the past fourteen months. On three days of that week, Pacheco brought people to look at the monkeys. The pictures too, he argued, were staged.

Following the raid, the police gave custody of the monkeys to Lori Kenealy of the local Humane Society, who kept them in the basement of her house. The monkeys were official evidence, and Taub and his lawyers demanded their return. Their request was granted by the court ten days after the raid. As mentioned by Peter Carlson in his *Washington Post* article, the monkeys suddenly disappeared from Kenealy's basement. According to Kenealy, she was not at home when they were taken and knew nothing about what had happened. PETA was then informed that Taub could not be prosecuted without the monkeys. In an unforeseen twist, the monkeys suddenly returned, their cages containing Spanish moss, which indicated they had been in Florida. The monkeys were given back to Taub, who carried out blood tests that revealed the monkeys were extremely stressed by their 2,000-mile trip and had developed transport fever.

After Taub's first trial, 113 out of the 119 charges against him were dismissed. He secured a second trial and was exculpated when the court ruled that Maryland's Prevention of Cruelty to Animals law did not apply to federally funded laboratories. About sixty-seven American professional societies made representations on his behalf to the NIH, which reversed its decision of withholding support. Taub was finally hired by the University of Alabama and received a grant to study stroke. There, he opened a clinic where he developed and practised his constraint-induced therapy.

In 1861, the French physician Paul Broca examined the brain of a man after his death. The man had only been able to produce sounds, with the lone recognizable word being 'tan'. On autopsy, Broca found a damaged area in the man's frontal lobe. He subsequently found damage in the same brain area in other people with similar speech problems. He thus localized the area of the brain responsible for speech. This area was later named Broca's area. Similarly, the entire human brain has been mapped. Each part of the body is assigned a specific motor and sensory region in the brain. This representation is called a cortical homunculus, Latin for 'little man'. This little man in the brain is, however, disproportionate to the big man, with huge hands, lips and face. The representation is thus not based on a region's surface area or volume but its function. For instance, the hands, which have more precise functions than the arms, have a larger region of the brain devoted to them than the arms do. This is the concept of anatomic localization.

The concept of neuroplasticity states that the brain has the ability to reorganize itself based on the stimuli it receives. It is a common observation that blind individuals have an increased sensitivity to touch and that some dancers who are deaf are still able to dance on beat as they can sense the vibrations produced by the speakers. The occipital region in the brain is the area responsible for vision, and when it stops receiving stimuli from the eyes, it can take up other functions by changing its various neuronal connections. Similarly, when an area of the brain is damaged, as in strokes, the surrounding area of the brain has the potential to reorganize itself by forming new connections to take over the function of the damaged segment.

Following Taub, many scientists began exploring the concept of neuroplasticity. The Silver Spring monkeys were viewed to be a valuable resource to prove this concept. Scientists wanted to study the neuroplastic changes that might have occurred in the brains of these monkeys after they were deprived of sensory inputs from their limbs for about twelve years following the deafferentation. The monkeys were in the custody of the NIH. As the monkeys grew old, they began to exhibit significant health issues. NIH scientists proposed one final set of experiments under deep anaesthesia, which was to be followed by the monkeys being euthanized. One of the monkeys was anaesthetized, a part of his skull was removed and electrodes were inserted in the sensory cortex area of the arm. When scientists stroked the monkey's arm, as expected, no signals were sent to the electrodes. But when they stroked the monkey's face, the neurons in the monkey's deafferented arm map began to fire, confirming that the facial map has taken over the arm map. This indicated brain reorganization over an area of 14 millimetres, the largest that had ever been mapped.

Thus, cortical reorganization in stroke patients can considerably improve their functional outcome. This can be achieved by consistently stimulating the brain by exercising the damaged limb and restraining the unaffected limb. The brain can recover as long as there is surrounding healthy tissue. Many people have benefitted from CIMT at Taub's clinic. Taub also developed a computerized version of this therapy, called AutoCITE, for people unable to visit his clinic. He also expanded his therapy to benefit individuals with other diseases, such as cerebral palsy or amyotrophic lateral sclerosis. His therapy has proven effective even for those who sought it years after their debilitating strokes.

Thinking inside the Box

The concept of 'learned paralysis' posits that the visual feedback of a limb's immobility after a stroke progressively reinforces the belief that the limb is incapable of movement. As the brain constantly sees that the limb does not move with the motor output sent to it, the representation of that limb in the sensory cortex progressively shrinks. The spared neurons for that region gradually reorganize and take over the function of the adjacent regions, and this leads to a further impairment of that limb.

This concept is different from Taub's 'learned non-use', which postulated that it was simply non-use that led to cortical reorganization. His therapeutic intervention was thus based on restricting the good arm. The therapy for learned paralysis, however, involves sending false visual feedback to the brain. The brain is shown and made to believe that the paralysed arm is functional again. This is achieved by using a mirror and a box.

Mirror therapy, or mirror visual feedback, was developed by the neuroscientist V.S. Ramachandran. It was originally devised to help people with phantom limb pain, a condition in which patients feel constant pain from an amputated limb, as if that limb were stuck in an uncomfortable position. A mirror box is a box with two mirrors in the centre, one facing each way. The patient positions the good limb on one side and the residual limb on the other. The patient then looks into the mirror on the good limb's side and attempts synchronized movements of both the limbs, such as trying to lift both the hands up. As the patient sees the reflection of the good hand moving, it appears as if the phantom hand is moving. Using this artificial feedback, the patient regains control over the phantom limb and is able to unclench it from the uncomfortable position, leading to an alleviation of the phantom pain.

It is important to note that the pain mechanisms are partially immune to intellectual correction. The individual with the phantom limb knows that the limb does not exist, yet experiences pain from it. The brain receives no visual signals that would contradict the pain. But when the patient looks at the visual reflection of the good arm in the mirror, as the optically resurrected phantom, the brain sees that there is no external object actually causing the pain, and thus rejects the pain as spurious.

The reflection of the working limb may thus stimulate movement in a weak or paralysed limb following a stroke. Just by looking at the mirror image of the good arm, the brain begins to form new neural connections and new pathways that help in the functional recovery of the paralysed limb.

The major advantage of this therapy is that it is easy to establish and can be practised at home. Various trials have shown that this technique is a powerful adjunct to conventional therapy.

Can't Talk, Yet Can Sing

Imagine a garden with two saplings planted side by side. As time passes, the sapling that receives more direct light grows into a far larger tree than the other and overshadows it. Consequently, the larger tree covers more space, while the other tree is much shorter, has fewer leaves and covers less area. Thus, the growth of one tree is effectively inhibited by the other tree. Now, if the bigger tree is cut, the smaller tree will have enough sunlight and space to grow to its full potential and would cover the whole area.

Our brains are composed of two hemispheres, the right and the left hemispheres, which are connected by a thick bundle of nerve fibres known as the corpus callosum. Both the hemispheres constantly interchange information through the corpus callosum. The left hemisphere controls the sensory and motor functions of the right side of the body, while the right hemisphere controls the left side of the body. One of the hemispheres is usually dominant over the other and sends inhibitory signals to it. In most individuals the left side is the dominant hemisphere. Some specialized functions are performed by only one hemisphere. For instance, only the left side has Broca's area, the area for speech.

Everything we think and do is due to the integrated efforts of both brain hemispheres. Both hemispheres receive sensory inputs separately and process these individually. If it weren't for the communication between the two hemispheres and the subsequent inhibition or stimulation of one by the other, it would be like two individuals living in one body. In some individuals with refractory epilepsy, the corpus callosum is surgically severed as a last resort for treatment when medications have failed, and this results in them having 'split-brain syndrome'. These individuals, however, appear normal, and their condition is apparent only with some special tests. In one such test, an individual with split-brain is made to look at a cross in the centre of a computer screen. Words flashed on the right side of the cross are seen by the left hemisphere, while words that appear to the left of the cross are seen by the right hemisphere. When the subject sees the image using the left hemisphere, they can identify and say what the word means. However, when it is seen by the right hemisphere, they are not able to say what the word means but can draw a picture of that word. The left hemisphere can then identify the picture and say what the word is. This demonstrates that the right hemisphere requires an external medium to communicate in the absence of the internal connection to the left hemisphere through the corpus callosum.

In very rare instances, individuals are born with only one hemisphere, as the other fails to develop at all. This might result from a haemorrhage while in the womb. However, these individuals can perform most functions and are only mildly impaired. A possible explanation is that as one hemisphere develops, it receives no interference from the other damaged side and has no inhibitory signals. Therefore, it assumes control of the entire body. These are the neuroplastic changes occurring in the earliest stages of life.

Following a stroke of the left hemisphere, individuals lose the ability to speak and thus communicate. Can neuroplasticity be used in these individuals to stimulate the other hemisphere to take over the function of speech? It turns out that while the area for speech is in the left hemisphere, the right hemisphere is responsible for processing music and rhythm. Therapists draw on this understanding to train individuals who lose their ability to talk following a stroke to sing instead. This therapy is known as melodic intonation therapy.

Stroke a Chord is a choir in Melbourne, Australia, comprised entirely of stroke victims who have lost the ability to talk. They are, however, able to sing due to the music processing ability of the right side of their brains.

Melodic intonation therapy is designed to lead an aphasic individual from intoning or singing two- to three-syllable phrases to saying more than five syllables across three levels of treatment. Each level introduces twenty high-probability words or social phrases presented with visual cues. Phrases are intonated on just two pitches and melodies are determined by the phrases' natural prosody. The therapist begins by humming a phrase shown by a visual cue and by tapping the patient's hand. They then sing the phrase while tapping the patient's hand. This is followed by the therapist and the patient singing the phrase together along with hand tapping. In the next step, the therapist fades away while the patient continues to sing the phrase, though hand tapping is continued. In the next step, the therapist first sings the phrase alone, and then the patient repeats it, assisted only by hand tapping. In the final step of this elementary level, the therapist intones a question and the patient answers by intoning the target phrase. Hand tapping is the only form of assistance, without any facial or visual cues.

As the therapy progresses from elementary to advanced, the phrases become more complex. For instance, a patient may start by singing, 'I love you', progress to singing, 'I love my children' in the intermediate level, and finally sing 'I love my son and daughter' in the advanced level.

Though this form of therapy has proven to be beneficial in the recovery of some language abilities, it requires a great deal of commitment in terms of time and resources, making it limited in its accessibility. A possible solution is to teach the patient's family members to administer this therapy at home.

NON-INVASIVE BRAIN STIMULATION

To understand the concept of non-invasive brain stimulation, consider a child with a disability being bullied at school. You could do two things: stop the bullying and encourage and provide support to the child being bullied. Non-invasive brain stimulation operates on the interhemispheric competition model. This suggests that functional recovery in stroke patients is hindered due to reduced output from the affected hemisphere and excessive inhibition by the unaffected hemisphere through the corpus callosum. Non-invasive stimulation involves the application of weak electric or magnetic fields to the brain via the surface of the scalp with the goal of changing or normalizing brain activity. The aim is to increase the excitability of the affected hemisphere and decrease the excitability of the opposite or unaffected hemisphere.

The two most common forms of non-invasive brain stimulation are transcranial magnetic stimulation (TMS) and transcranial direct current stimulation (tDCS). TMS uses a rapidly changing magnetic field to induce electric currents in the brain and stimulate the neurons. In tDCS, a small battery-powered device is used to deliver weak electric currents (usually 1–2 mA) to the brain via saline-soaked sponges placed over the stimulation site. Depending upon the technique used, an increase or decrease in brain activity is achieved by altering the frequency at which the stimulation is performed, changing the pattern of stimulation or reversing the polarity of the electrodes. Both TMS and tDCS are not only safe and effective in changing brain activity but they also enhance motor adaptation, learning and motor memory consolidation in both healthy adults and stroke survivors.

STROKE AND DEPRESSION

Depression is one of the most important yet frequently overlooked complication of stroke. About 30 per cent of stroke patients experience depression. Patients can develop new personality traits due to damage in certain areas of the brain. They may become apathetic, inflexible, rigid, impulsive, insensitive or indifferent to others; adopt a poor perception of self; or become guilt-ridden, paranoid or even suicidal.

The root cause of these emotional shifts remains unclear. They could stem from the loss in ability that patients feel or from brain damage itself, which can cause a depletion of certain chemicals called neurotransmitters that affect mood.

The repercussions of a stroke extend beyond the patient, affecting the whole family. Those with severe deficits often become dependent on caregivers for daily activities and physical and emotional support. The caregivers can themselves develop feelings of entrapment, isolation, anger or depression.

Thus, along with pharmacological therapy to treat depression, it is important for physicians to provide psychological support and encouragement to both stroke patients and their family members, recognizing the toll a stroke can take.

12

Stroke in the Young

Children are not only innocent and curious but also optimistic and joyful and essentially happy. They are, in short, everything adults wish they could be.

—Carolyn Haywood

THE BEST CHILDREN'S hospital in the United States is the Boston Children's Hospital (BCH). It was founded in July 1869 by Dr Francis Henry Brown, a Civil War surgeon, who travelled to Europe in 1867 to study the pioneering field of paediatrics. Brown was impressed with the treatments he witnessed and wanted to bring that level of care to children in Boston. Along with the city's civic leaders and a small group of graduates from Harvard Medical School that he put together, Brown established a children's hospital in a townhouse on Rutland Street in Boston's South End. Although it had a capacity of twenty beds, the hospital treated thirty patients in its inaugural year. One year later, the hospital relocated to a larger building on the same street. Most patients were from the Irish immigrant community, and many had traumatic injuries or infectious diseases. The hospital was largely supported by many philanthropists. For the first forty-five years of its existence, Sister Theresa and the Anglican Order of the Sisters of St. Margaret oversaw the nursing care of the children in the hospital.

By 1882, the hospital moved to a larger building on Huntington Avenue. Between 1882 and 1914, the practice of paediatrics was recognized as a speciality, and Harvard Medical School made its first appointment of a physician devoted solely to the care of children. Harvard Medical School affiliated itself with BCH in 1903. In the early 1900s, Harvard Medical School moved to its current site, and in 1914, BCH relocated to its current address on Longwood Avenue, adjacent to the Medical School. Various sub-specialities were subsequently developed, such as surgery, medicine, radiology and orthopaedics. Surgeons developed new techniques to repair congenital abnormalities (birth defects). The field of cardiac surgery began and the iron lung for polio victims was developed by physicians at BCH and the Harvard School of Public Health. Harvard medical students began to learn paediatrics at BCH. The house staff grew from three to four in 1900 and to over thirty in the early '40s. As men left to serve in World War II, more women were recruited as residents.

Currently, the hospital's research enterprise is larger than any other paediatric medical centre in the world. Its discoveries, whether they were in terms of recognition of diseases, or the development of medical and surgical treatments, have benefitted children and adults since 1869, some of which are worth mentioning here.

By 1891, milk from infected cows was recognized as a common source of disease among poor children. Thomas Morgan Rotch, BCH's chief physician, established the nation's first laboratory for the modification and production of bacteria-free milk.

In 1920, Dr William Ladd launched the speciality of paediatric surgery by devising procedures to correct various birth defects. The era of modern paediatric cardiac surgery began in 1938, when Dr Robert E. Gross performed the world's first successful surgical procedure to correct a congenital heart defect. In 1986, BCH's surgeons performed the hospital's first heart transplant.

Dr Sidney Farber, a paediatric pathologist, conducted trials on children with leukemia (a type of blood cancer), a diagnosis that was deemed a death sentence in 1948. He achieved the world's first partial remission of acute leukemia. He went on to co-found the Dana–Farber Cancer Institute in 1950. In 1971, Dr Judah Folkman published the first paper that described the theory that tumours recruit new blood vessels to grow. BCH's chief of haematology and oncology, David Nathan, recommended hydroxyurea, a drug used to treat blood cancer, to a patient with sickle cell disease. The treatment worked, and hydroxyurea is now broadly used to treat sickle cell disease.

In 1949, Dr John Enders, his assistant Thomas Weller and his colleague Frederick Robbins successfully cultured the polio virus, making possible the development of polio vaccines by Jonas Salk and Albert Bruce Sabin. They won the Nobel Prize for their work in 1954. Enders and his team then went on to culture the measles virus.

In 1972, the Boston brace, a new brace for patients with scoliosis, was developed by Chief of Orthopaedics John E. Hall and orthotist Bill Miller. In the same decade, BCH conducted a widespread study on donated teeth from children and measured the lead levels in those teeth. The results showed that children with higher levels of lead in their teeth were far behind those with lower levels on measures including IQ, motor coordination and attentiveness in the classroom.

∽

Child neurology as an independent field developed with the Department of Neurology at Boston Children's Hospital. The history of the department is really the history of the field of child neurology. It was founded in 1929 by Dr Bronson Crothers as 'Ward 9', the first dedicated space for child neurology at a US children's hospital. Crothers went on to make landmark contributions to the study of cerebral palsy. My time at Ward 9 as a visiting medical student is one of my most treasured experiences. I was astonished by the complexities of neurological diseases and, at the same time, by the advancements at BCH.

The first comprehensive paediatric seizure unit in the world was established at BCH. The epilepsy centre remains at the forefront of paediatric epilepsy care and research to this day. Within child neurology many subspeciality programs run at BCH, such as brain tumour, headache, tuberous sclerosis, Sturge–Weber syndrome, Rett syndrome, stroke, brain injury/concussion, autism, neuroimmunology/multiple sclerosis, movement disorders and spinal muscular atrophy.

Dr Michael Rivkin founded and directs the Stroke and Cerebrovascular Center at BCH. This centre provides care for children who suffer from stroke, with clinicians in the disciplines of neurology, haematology, psychiatry, neuropsychology, neuroradiology, neurosurgery, interventional neuroradiology, occupational therapy and physical therapy. The centre also offers a fellowship programme to train paediatric neurologists to evaluate and care for children who have suffered strokes or have cerebrovascular disorders.

I first met Dr Rivkin at one of the weekly neuroradiology conferences held at BCH. I expressed my interest in stroke, and he arranged for me to spend time in his department the following week. Prior to this, I did not have a lot of knowledge of paediatric stroke. After attending the clinics, I realized how different paediatric stroke is from adult stroke. The causes of stroke in children, their presentation and treatment approaches are not the same as in adults.

That one week was an enlightening experience. I not only gained a lot of knowledge about stroke but also learnt a lot from the patients I interacted with. While adults tend to focus on their disabilities, the children focused on their abilities. I have a lot of respect and admiration for these young fighters and their families.

About 65 per cent of strokes occur after the age of sixty-five, which means 35 per cent occur before it. Although strokes and damage from vascular disease are by far most common in adults and the elderly, strokes occur at all ages, including neonates, babies, young children, adolescents and young adults. Annualized paediatric stroke incidence rates, including both neonatal and later childhood and both ischemic and haemorrhagic stroke, range from three to twenty-five per 100,000 children in developed countries.

There are different ways of categorizing paediatric stroke. One is by age: stroke occurring from twenty-eight weeks of gestation (inside the womb) to twenty-eight days postnatal (after birth) is classified as perinatal stroke. Stroke occurring between twenty-eight days and eighteen years of age is classified as childhood stroke.

Sometimes perinatal stroke is detected at the time it occurs because the infant will present with focal seizures and encephalopathy. Then there is presumed stroke—where the stroke is presumed to have occurred in the perinatal period but the diagnosis is made later, when infants present with various symptoms. For example, children usually develop a preferential use of one hand by the age of eighteen months, but if an infant is showing early handedness or an early preference of one hand over the other, they might need brain imaging, which could show a remote stroke. Some of these children with presumed perinatal ischemic stroke may have had clinical or subclinical seizures that escaped detection in the neonatal period because of the challenges of distinguishing neonatal seizures from normal infant movements.

Perinatal stroke can be either ischaemic or haemorrhagic, resulting from disruptions of either arteries or veins from early gestation through the first month of life. An MRI is employed to diagnose the stroke. Magnetic resonance angiography (MRA) and magnetic resonance venography (MRV) are performed when venous thrombosis is suspected.

Brain haemorrhages in newborns also have non-specific findings. The causes of brain haemorrhage in term neonates include disorders in the coagulation system, low platelet count, trauma and rarely, structural abnormalities in the blood vessels of the brain. Although no specific cause can be identified in the majority of neonates with haemorrhagic stroke, risk factors include postmaturity, emergency caesarean delivery, foetal distress and male sex. The neonatal brain has little capability to autoregulate according to blood pressure and blood flow, so it is more vulnerable to falls or elevations in blood pressure, and as a result the arteries rupture easily with increased blood pressure.

An effective way to decrease the incidence of haemorrhages in newborns is vitamin K administration. A single injection of vitamin K in the muscle of a newborn can prevent bleeding in many cases. This practice has become a routine procedure at births all over the world, and it benefits thousands of infants annually. Vitamin K converts the clotting factors II, VII, IX and X into an active state. A deficiency of vitamin K leads to inadequate activity of these clotting factors, which results in bleeding. Being a fat-soluble vitamin, it is mainly synthesized in adults by the bacteria present in the gut. Newborns have minimal vitamin K reserves in their liver and are not able to synthesize vitamin K due to the absence of bacteria in their gut. Hence, they are more prone to bleeding in their skin, gut and brain. Bleeding due to vitamin K deficiency can occur anywhere between the first week of birth till three months, but it mostly presents in the first week. Since breast milk is not a good source of vitamin K, babies who are exclusively breastfed may develop a deficiency. Additionally, babies whose mothers ingested drugs such as warfarin, phenytoin or barbiturates during pregnancy sometimes develop bleeding related to vitamin K deficiency.

In children, the presentation of stroke is similar to those in adults. The most common symptoms include loss of function in one side of the body or weakness in one side of the face, speech or language disturbance, vision disturbance and difficulty walking. Children sometimes present with non-specific symptoms such as headaches and altered mental status. Seizures at stroke onset are more common in children than in adults. Clinical presentation varies according to age, setting (inpatient versus emergency department) and stroke subtype.

Because strokes are relatively less common in children than in adults, there is often a delay in diagnosing a child with stroke. The major causes of delays include delayed consideration of stroke among frontline providers and delays in accessing MRI, often because children need sedation or anaesthesia to remain still in the MRI machine. Only about 60 per cent of children with strokes are accurately diagnosed by emergency medical providers, giving 40 per cent an incorrect initial diagnosis of stroke mimics. Stroke mimics are other neurological conditions that have a similar clinical presentation as a stroke. The most common are migraine with aura, Bell's palsy and seizures, especially with Todd's paresis. Other stroke mimics include brain tumours, infections, traumatic brain injury, intoxication, metabolic disease and psychogenic disorders.

Brain haemorrhages, injuries, infections and birth defects in the heart are significant causes of stroke in children, adolescents and young adults. In preadolescent children, malformations of the brain blood vessels are the most common cause of bleeding. Before the age of twenty, subarachnoid haemorrhages due to ruptured aneurysms are a slightly more common cause of bleeding than vascular malformations.

The major causes of brain ischemia in children are embolisms from the heart, dissections of the arteries, thrombosis of dural sinuses and veins, coagulation abnormalities and arteriopathies.

Common risk factors for adult ischemic strokes, such as hypertension, diabetes, increased blood cholesterols and smoking, play a diminished role in childhood brain ischemia. About a quarter of ischemic strokes in young children are attributable to heart disease. Brain infarcts in children with heart disease are most often caused by embolism. Infection of the heart valves (bacterial endocarditis) and complex birth defects are major causes. Children with heart defects are often in a state of low oxygen due to a mixing of venous blood (low-oxygen blood returning to the heart) and arterial blood (oxygen-rich blood pumped to the body by the left side of the heart). In order to compensate for low blood oxygen levels, the red blood cells in the body increase in number, a phenomenon known as polycythemia. This surge in blood cells can block arteries and veins, leading to strokes.

Arterial composition and function in children are different from that in most adults, since they are rarely subjected to atherosclerosis. Arteriopathy in this group develops from a number of other stimuli. Arteriopathies are characterized by local and generalized regions of narrowing, occlusion or dilation of large arteries in the brain. They have a variety of different causes, including infection, trauma, migraine, moyamoya disease and genetic conditions such as sickle cell disease, Fabry disease and mitochondrial disorders.

Moyamoya disease is a condition of unknown cause that develops in children and young adults. In cases of moyamoya, the internal carotid arteries in the skull gradually become occluded. The reduction in blood flow in these major vessels of the anterior circulation of the brain leads to a compensatory development of collateral vasculature by small vessels near the apex of the carotid, on the cortical surface, leptomeninges, and branches of the external carotid artery supplying the dura and the base of the skull. In rare cases, this process also involves the posterior circulation, including the basilar and posterior cerebral arteries.

When moyamoya was first described in 1957, it was termed 'hypoplasia of bilateral internal carotid arteries'. The characteristic appearance of the associated network of abnormally dilated collateral vessels on angiographies was later likened to 'something hazy, like a puff of cigarette smoke'. This description translates to 'moyamoya' in Japanese. Moyamoya is the most common paediatric cerebrovascular disease in Japan, with a prevalence of approximately three cases per 100,000 children. As a result, moyamoya was originally considered to predominantly affect those of Asian heritage. It has now been observed throughout the world in people of many ethnic backgrounds, including American and European populations. It typically manifests in two age groups: children around the age of five and adults in their mid-forties. Moyamoya can present in children as seizures, headache or ischemic or haemorrhagic strokes.

Sickle cell disease is a group of inherited red blood cell disorders that affects haemoglobin, the protein that carries oxygen throughout the body. Normally, red blood cells are disc-shaped and flexible, so that they can move easily through the blood vessels. But in sickle cell disease, the red blood cells are crescent- or sickle-shaped. These cells do not bend and move easily, and they can block blood flow to the rest of the body. This blocked blood flow can lead to strokes, eye problems, infections and episodes of pain, called pain crises. These patients require regular blood transfusions or hydroxyurea for prevention and treatment.

Arteriopathy can also arise from trauma. The stretching of arteries at locations where they are not anchored can lead to the tearing of arterial walls (dissections). Even trivial neck traumas can injure children's arteries. Young children may fall while holding objects like pencils or toothbrushes in their mouths, injuring or lacerating the pharynx and internal carotid artery, which runs behind the tonsillar pillars in the throat. Carotid and vertebral artery dissections in the neck can develop after head or neck injuries, especially involving sudden twisting movements (rollercoaster rides) or blunt trauma to the neck. Bow Hunter's syndrome, named for the turning of the head when using a bow as an archer, is an uncommon cause of vertebrobasilar insufficiency that results from occlusion or injury to the vertebral artery during neck rotation. The cause is often a bony abnormality that may compress the vertebral artery, compromising blood flow or leading to vessel wall injury, resulting in thromboembolism.

Infections can also cause strokes in children. The internal carotid artery in the neck lies close to the tonsils, and an infection of the tonsils can cause its occlusion. Influenza, Mycoplasma pneumoniae, enteroviruses, HIV and spirochetes that cause Lyme disease and syphilis are other known causes of stroke. Varicella-zoster virus (VZV) causes chicken pox in children and shingles or herpes zoster in adults. This virus attacks the nerves and the blood vessels. It gains access to the brain arteries by way of the meninges and through nerves that innervate the arteries. If the virus infects the wall of a blood vessel, it can cause thrombosis by activating platelets and triggering blood clot formation, a process described in Virchow's triad.

Lastly, migraines are also common in children with strokes. It is theorized that migraines might cause strokes either by causing prolonged constriction of blood vessels or by prompting the formation of local thrombi related to vascular narrowing and activation of the clotting system. Children's blood vessels are more prone than adults.

※

In young adults between the ages of twenty to forty, atherosclerosis is a much less common cause of stroke than in older age groups. However, high blood pressure, diabetes, smoking or high levels of cholesterol can lead to premature atherosclerosis and strokes among young adults. The significant causes of stroke in adults under forty include bleeding due to tearing of the blood vessel wall, clots from the heart, abnormal connections between arteries and veins, clots in large veins (sinuses), the use of illicit drugs, pregnancy-related complications and other systemic illnesses. Frequent athletic activities and vigorous exercises, and the mobility of youthful arteries can lead to their tearing. Mobile arteries are more readily torn during sudden or extreme head and neck movements, or with trauma.

Illicit drug use, a plague among adolescents and young adults, continues to be a frequent cause of strokes. Amphetamines usually lead to brain haemorrhages, while cocaine can cause both haemorrhagic and ischemic strokes. Heroin and drugs packaged for oral use but injected intravenously can cause strokes by blocking the arteries.

There is a small increase in the risk of stroke during pregnancy and the postpartum period and when taking pills containing female hormones. Eclampsia, characterized by very high blood pressure during pregnancy, is the most frequent cause of stroke in these women. Heart disease and other conditions present before pregnancy can also promote strokes during pregnancy and the postpartum period.

In many young adults, strokes are directly related to systemic conditions and infections. Cancer and leukemia affect blood clotting and can cause both ischemic and haemorrhagic strokes. Some infections directly or indirectly affect the blood vessels inside the head. Tuberculosis, syphilis and cysticercosis (contracted by ingesting pork tapeworm eggs) are examples of infections that can cause brain ischemia. Bacterial endocarditis, an infection of the heart valves, can result in strokes due to the embolization of infectious materials that create a vegetation on the surface of the valves. In patients with HIV/AIDS, enhanced clotting can develop and superimposed infections can directly affect brain blood vessels. Many inflammatory conditions, such as Crohn's disease, ulcerative colitis and rheumatoid arthritis, can cause enhanced clotting and lead to thrombosis of the arteries and veins in the head. Systemic lupus erythematous, a condition that is most prevalent in young women, leads to strokes by causing heart valve lesions and blood abnormalities.

Given the multitude of potential causes for strokes and cerebrovascular abnormalities in children and young adults, diagnostic evaluations and tests are often more extensive and diverse than in the elderly.

13

Genes

Genes are like the story, and DNA is the language that the story is written in.

—Sam Kean

CADASIL AND CARASIL

IN 1976, A fifty-year-old man arrived at the University of Paris after experiencing a minor stroke. Unusually, he presented no risk factors that could cause a stroke at his age. His CT scan showed multiple strokes in the small arteries of the brain. These small strokes were confirmed ten years later on an MRI, which had become available by then. The absence of any risk factors made the diagnosis unclear, so the patient's doctors had to settle on a diagnosis of Binswanger's disease.

However, Marie-Germaine Bousser, an assistant neurologist assigned to the case, was not convinced by this diagnosis. In order to keep an eye on the patient, she enrolled him in one of the first aspirin prevention clinical trials in stroke patients. The patient remained under observation until his death twenty years later. He had progressively developed difficulty in walking and memory impairment. Notably, during this period, the patient's two children, both in their thirties, were also diagnosed with minor strokes. Their MRIs showed similarities to their father's. This led to the hypothesis of a hereditary condition.

Bousser discussed these three unusual cases of familial stroke with a fellow neurologist, Elisabeth Tournier-Lasserve, who had a growing interest in the research being done in this field. They collaborated and began their own research in 1990. They planned to investigate all the consenting relatives of the first three clinical cases through detailed clinical examination, MRI and DNA extraction. Owing to the willingness of the whole family, as many as fifty-seven adult members were evaluated. It was confirmed that the disease was genetic, an autosomal dominant condition affecting the small arteries and capillaries in the brain. (An autosomal dominant condition is when only a single copy of an abnormal gene is required from either parent to cause a disease. In autosomal recessive diseases two copies of an abnormal gene, one from each parent, are required to cause disease.)

In 1993, the data obtained from the study of this family allowed the gene locus of the disease to be assigned to chromosome 19q12, which was confirmed immediately in a second French family. The label 'cerebral autosomal dominant arteriopathy with subcortical infarcts and leukoencephalopathy' (CADASIL) was given by Bousser to designate the disease.

They expanded their research and recruited thirty-two additional French families with CADASIL to participate in the study and collaborated with two other young neurologists.

Tournier-Lasserve welcomed Anne Joutel, who had recently completed a residency with Bousser, into her lab to pivot into the basic sciences so as to identify the mutation. Huges Chabriat, who had also trained with Bousser, became the group's expert on the clinical aspects of CADASIL. Joutel and Tournier-Lasserve subsequently identified the responsible gene as NOTCH3, a gene that had previously only been studied in fruit flies.

CADASIL is the most commonly inherited small artery disease of the brain. Prior to its discovery, almost 30 per cent of patients with CADASIL used to be diagnosed with multiple sclerosis and had to undergo immunosuppressive therapy. Many other patients were diagnosed with psychiatric disorders and institutionalized in psychiatric facilities.

The most common presentation of CADASIL is recurrent small strokes around the mean age of forty-nine, in patients who generally do not have any other risk factors for stroke. Other manifestations include decline in cognitive function, migraines with aura, mood disturbances and severe depression.

The discovery of CADASIL opened the doors for the discovery of several other genes affecting the small blood vessels in the brain.

Cerebral autosomal recessive arteriopathy with subcortical infarcts and leukoencephalopathy (CARASIL) is a rare autosomal recessive disease affecting the small arteries in the brain. The term was proposed by Bowler and Hachinski, based on the disorder's recessive inheritance and resemblance to CADASIL. A very small number of cases of CARASIL have been described across the globe. Most of them have been diagnosed in Japan, with a few additional cases reported in Chinese, Turkish, Spanish and Romanian patients. In addition to small strokes, CARASIL patients present with memory impairment at an early age, difficulty in walking, hair loss and lower back pain.

∽

Sickle Cell Disease

Sickle cell disease refers to a group of inherited blood disorders, the most common type being sickle cell anaemia. It affects haemoglobin, the protein that carries oxygen throughout the body. The condition impacts more than 100,000 people in the United States and twenty million people worldwide.

I first learnt about sickle cell disease in pre-med while studying genetics in biology. It serves as a classic example of how a single base substitution in DNA can lead to an abnormal protein. We were then taught about it in biochemistry in the first year of medical school, then again in pathology, pharmacology and microbiology in our second year and then in medicine during the final year.

In healthy individuals, red blood cells are disc-shaped and flexible so that they can move easily through the blood vessels. But in sickle cell disease, a single base substitution from GAG to GUG at the sixth codon of the beta globin results in the substitution of glutamic acid by valine at the sixth position of the beta globin chain of the haemoglobin molecule. Due to this abnormal haemoglobin, the red blood cells become crescent- or sickle-shaped under certain conditions such as stress, dehydration, temperature changes or high altitude. These cells do not bend and move easily, and they can block the blood flow to the rest of the body. This blocked blood flow throughout the body can lead to serious problems, such as strokes, eye problems, infections and episodes of pain. The blood vessels can be blocked anywhere in the body. When in the brain, they lead to strokes, and when in the chest, they lead to acute chest syndrome.

The first description of sickle cell disease was given by James Herrick, a cardiologist practising in Chicago, in 1910. The patient was a twenty-year-old dental student from the island of Grenada in the Caribbean. He developed what is now called acute chest syndrome and was admitted to the Presbyterian Hospital in Chicago, where he was monitored by an intern, Ernest Irons, and his attending physician, Herrick. Irons saw 'peculiar elongated and sickle-shaped' cells in the patient's blood. The second case, published only three months later, was a twenty-five-year-old woman who had been observed for some years in the wards of the Medical College of Virginia. The third case that was reported was a twenty-one-year-old woman with a characteristic blood film. The fresh blood film obtained from the father of this patient was normal, but when the blood preparation was sealed and observed days later, there were similarly abnormal red cells. The authors inferred that sickling of the red blood cells might be an inherited phenomenon. The fourth case, a twenty-one-year-old man, reported from Johns Hopkins Hospital, was the first in which the term 'sickle cell anemia' was used. Memphis physician Lemuel Diggs first introduced the distinction between sickle cell disease and sickle cell trait in 1933.

In November 1949, Linus Carl Pauling, Harvey Itano, S.J. Singer and Ibert Wells published 'Sickle Cell Anemia, a Molecular Disease' in the journal *Science*. It reported the first piece of evidence of a human disease being caused by an abnormal protein. Sickle cell anaemia became the first disease understood at the molecular level. Using electrophoresis, they demonstrated that individuals with sickle cell disease had a modified form of haemoglobin in their red blood cells and that patients with sickle cell trait had both the normal and abnormal forms of haemoglobin. This was the first demonstration casually linking an abnormal protein to a disease and also the first demonstration showing that Mendelian inheritance determined the specific physical properties of proteins, not simply their presence or absence, cementing the foundation of molecular genetics.

In 1956, Vernon Ingram determined that the change in the haemoglobin molecule in sickle cell disease and trait was the substitution of the glutamic acid in position six of the beta chain of the normal protein by valine. Ingram used electrophoresis and chromatography to demonstrate that the amino acid sequence of normal human and sickle cell anaemia haemoglobins differed due to a single substituted amino acid residue. This was the first time a researcher showed that a single amino acid exchange in a protein could cause a disease or a condition. As a result, Vernon Ingram is often referred to as the 'father of molecular medicine'.

There are several other genetic disorders that can lead to strokes along with many other manifestations. An exhaustive dissection of each disorder is, unfortunately, beyond the scope of the book.

There are some abnormal genes that can directly lead to strokes, and then there are those that can increase the risk of and susceptibility to conventional stroke risk factors, such as hypertension, atrial fibrillation and diabetes. They influence specific mechanisms underlying strokes, such as the occurrence and progression of atherosclerosis. They can also create a predisposition to clot formation or bleeding and modify the brain's resilience to injury.

Popular genetic research methods include candidate gene studies and genome-wide association studies (GWAS). The candidate gene approach to conducting genetic association studies focuses on associations between genetic variation within pre-specified genes of interest and disease states. The approach is limited by its reliance on existing knowledge about known or theoretical biology of disease. The results with candidate gene studies in stroke have not been very promising, and the genomic analysis of stroke has shifted to GWAS.

The development of accurate and high-throughput technologies using microarrays has made it possible to analyse the entire genome (complete set of genes) of a study subject. This has led to GWAS, which consists of genotyping a very large number of genetic variations and testing their associations with disease states without any prior hypothesis or underlying biology. GWAS has led to many significant associations of genetic variations to stroke.

The study of stroke genetics required large collaborative efforts and led to the creation of international consortia. The International Stroke Genetics Consortium (ISGC) was founded in April 2007 by Jonathan Rosand, a professor of neurology at Harvard, endowed chair in neurology at Massachusetts General Hospital (MGH) and an associate member of the Broad Institute in Cambridge, Massachusetts. He convened the founding members—sixteen investigators from Europe and North America—at the Broad Institute. He then served as chair of the ISGC from 2007 through 2010 and the inaugural chair of the ISGC steering committee when it was created in 2011.

His laboratory continued to support the ISGC convener. He launched the ISGC's Cerebrovascular Disease Knowledge Portal. His research group at the MGH Center for Genomic Medicine and at the Broad Institute served as a training ground for many researchers who later developed internationally distinguished research programmes of their own.

The ISGC has been at the forefront of genetic discovery to understand stroke mechanisms. Its core values include collaboration and coordinated effort to produce effective results. The ISGC has developed other major stroke collaborations, including the METASTROKE consortium and the SiGN consortium, and has partnered with the CHARGE consortium. The ISGC has grown substantially, encompassing over 250 members from six continents spanning more than fifty countries. There have been multiple publications from the data derived from the ISGC. The first ISGC workshop was held in London in July 2007. Since then, it has held its international workshop every six months.

14

Prevention Is Better than Cure

> *The doctor of the future will give no medication, but will interest his patients in the care of the human frame, diet and in the cause and prevention of disease.*
>
> —Thomas A. Edison

> *When meditating over a disease, I never think of finding a remedy for it, but, instead, a means of preventing it.*
>
> —Louis Pasteur

> *He who cures a disease may be the skillfullest, but he that prevents it is the safest physician.*
>
> —Thomas Fuller

> *Intellectuals solve problems—geniuses prevent them.*
>
> —Albert Einstein

PREVENTION OFFERS US all a greater likelihood of benefit against strokes than even the most effective treatments.

While concerted efforts by the medical community and the media have been relatively successful in educating the public on heart attacks, cancer and AIDS, the general understanding of stroke remains limited.

During my third year of medical school, as part of our community medicine training, we undertook a project to gauge the public's awareness of strokes. In order to do this, we designed a questionnaire that asked whether they knew about the risk factors related to stroke, how stroke occurs and what they would do if they saw someone having a stroke. Organized in groups, we would travel to the rural areas around our institute to verbally ask people these questions and then record their responses.

The findings were revealing. Most people did not know that stroke involved the brain. A lay person views stroke as a paralysis of the arm or leg. They do not know that it is a blood vessel in the brain that is affected and that the impairment of the part of the brain controlling an arm or leg leads to its paralysis. Some people still believe stroke to be a punishment from God and resort to faith healing. We asked people what they'd do if someone around them experienced a stroke. Some suggested they would make the person 'smell a shoe' or give them *afeem*, which is opium (once called 'God's own medicine'). In certain less-educated pockets of India, the act of smelling a shoe has been a popular remedy for both epilepsy and stroke. Unfortunately, these treatments have no proven benefit and the patient loses the critical time window for medical treatment that can possibly reverse the deficiency. As a result, even when treatment is within their reach, most people fail to recognize its need and end up with permanent disabilities.

A stroke can be prevented by recognizing the risk factors, and permanent disability can be prevented by first recognizing its onset symptoms and then seeking timely treatment.

Heart attacks occur when the blood vessels in the heart are affected, and strokes occur when the blood vessels in the brain are affected. The risk factors for the two are thus the same, and the means to prevent them are also similar. These include good eating habits, regular exercise and avoidance of alcohol and cigarettes. Managing high blood pressure, diabetes and high cholesterol helps diminish the risk for both heart disease and stroke.

HYPERTENSION

High blood pressure is the single most important modifiable risk factor for stroke. It is associated with a two- to three-fold increase in the risk of stroke and accounts for almost a third of stroke risk. High blood pressure is very common—many individuals over the age of sixty have it. Several studies have shown that hypertension is underrecognized and undertreated, and numerous individuals with hypertension remain either undiagnosed or inadequately treated. Elevated blood pressure causes wear and tear in the blood vessels that supply the brain with blood. Chronic high blood pressure causes the thickening of arteries and leads to atherosclerosis and the narrowing of arteries.

Regular exercise and a healthy diet can reduce elevated blood pressure. In overweight individuals, weight loss can reduce blood pressure substantially. Decreasing alcohol intake and reducing salt consumption also help. Birth control pills have been shown to elevate blood pressure in some women, and stopping these pills can bring the pressure down. Various drugs are available to reduce blood pressure, and they are tailored for each individual and monitored by doctors to determine their effectiveness.

DIABETES

Diabetes is another important risk factor for stroke. Diabetes has a hereditary component: when both parents have diabetes, the development of diabetes in their children is almost certain. The last twenty years have seen a diabetes epidemic of sorts. This is driven partly by increased frequency of diagnosis and by a growing portion of the population being overweight or, in extreme cases, obese.

A Victorian-era physician described diabetes as 'one of the penalties of advanced civilization'. Diabetes was considered to be a product of wealth, dietary change and urbanization.

Interestingly, much of the evidence that diabetes was a disease of the rich came from India. At a meeting on tropical diabetes in 1907, it was said that 'what gout is to the nobility of England, diabetes is to the aristocracy of India' and 'exercise, as a rule, is disliked by the gentlemen class of Bengal after a certain age'. The 'Bengali babu' (a clerk who could write English) consumed excessive starches and sugars and had a completely sedentary lifestyle. His girth had a tendency to increase in direct proportion to an increment in his pay. By contrast, diabetes was almost unknown among Hindu widows, who led an unexciting life and did not consume any excess of sugars or other delicacies.

Elliott Proctor Joslin was the first doctor in the United States to specialize in diabetes and was the founder of Joslin Diabetes

Center. Found in the Longwood Medical Area, Boston, and affiliated with Harvard Medical School, it is the world's largest diabetes research centre, diabetes clinic and provider of diabetes education.

Joslin was the first to make a reference to an epidemic of diabetes in 1921. He talked about one in his hometown of Oxford, Massachusetts. Six out of seven people in adjoining houses had died of diabetes, and he pointed out that had they died of cholera, the public health authorities would have been around like a shot. But because it was diabetes, nobody was particularly bothered. In the 1930s, Joslin worked with the Metropolitan Life Insurance Company and established that the main risk factor for diabetes was being overweight. He noted that environmental conditions were also partly reported. The rapid use of machines lightened the burden of farm workers and transferred them into clerical and sales jobs, reducing the hours of labour. The amount of energy expended in manual work was drastically reduced for a majority of the working population.

The diet of our Palaeolithic ancestors was very different from ours. A third of the food consumed by the hunter-gatherers would have been protein with a very low-fat content, resulting in a more muscular and fit physique. Their carbohydrate intake would have varied but was likely fibre-rich. They would also, in common with all other mammals, have ingested more potassium than sodium. This is relevant because a high salt or sodium intake is one of the key factors leading to high blood pressure.

Despite the vast differences in time and lifestyle, modern humans still have the same Palaeolithic genotype, and in those who adhere to a traditional lifestyle today, diabetes and hypertension are rare. Individuals who have a high salt intake and high-energy diet and who do not exercise face a different story. And society leans towards this lifestyle—over the decades, portion sizes have increased. Between the 1970s and the 1990s, a typical snack increased from 160 to 250 calories and a soft drink from 130 to 200.

The two most recognized forms of diabetes mellitus are type 1 and type 2. Type 1 diabetes is caused by an insulin deficiency, and patients with this type of diabetes need to inject themselves with insulin. Type 1 diabetes often develops in childhood or during early adult life. Type 2 diabetes usually develops in adulthood and is most common in overweight individuals. Unlike people with type 1 diabetes, these individuals produce insulin, but the insulin does not use blood sugar efficiently for energy. Type 2 diabetes is often managed by dietary changes and pills that help lower blood sugar.

Individuals at risk for diabetes must carefully watch their weight and should follow a well-rounded diet that is relatively low in calories, carbohydrates and salt.

ABNORMALITIES OF BLOOD LIPIDS AND HIGH CHOLESTEROL

High cholesterol levels promote the formation of plaque in the arteries supplying the heart, limbs and brain. Cholesterol and other lipids circulate in the blood attached to lipoproteins. There are two main types of lipoproteins in the blood: HDL, which is also known as good cholesterol, and LDL, which is called bad cholesterol. High levels of LDL and low levels of HDL are risk factors for stroke and heart disease. Individuals who have family members with high cholesterol are more likely than others to develop high blood cholesterol. It is important for them to recognize lipid abnormalities and know their levels of cholesterol and other blood lipids early in life. High cholesterol can effectively be lowered with a healthy diet, exercise and medication. There are many medications to lower lipids, and some have more effects on certain lipid elements than others. They are usually tailored according to the needs of the patient, and sometimes a combination of drugs is used.

Medications like statins, used to lower cholesterol, have additional functions that can limit the risk of strokes. Statins have an effect on the lining of blood vessels—they limit the formation of atherosclerotic plaque. Even when blood cholesterol is normal, statins can prevent the build-up of plaque and may even reduce its size. Some physicians prescribe statin drugs for patients with strokes and for individuals with plaque who have not yet had strokes to reduce plaque development and enhance plaque reabsorption. Statins may also have a protective effect on the brain, increasing its resistance to reductions in blood flow.

Dr Caplan always advised his patients to take statins at night to decrease the absorption of lipids eaten during the day. One side effect of statins is that they can cause cramping and discomfort, but serious muscle injury is quite rare, occurring in less than 1 per cent of cases.

TRANSIENT ISCHEMIC ATTACKS

When someone experiences a sudden weakness in their arm or leg; a numbness of the face, arm or leg; a temporary loss of vision in one eye; double vision; an inability to speak normally; incoordination of the limbs or imbalance when walking; or dizziness and loss of balance, it's easy to dismiss these signs if they last only a few minutes. These symptoms are caused by the same vascular problems that cause strokes. These are known as transient ischemic attacks (TIAs).

TIAs indicate a problem in the arteries. When the lack of blood flow is brief or relatively minor, temporary loss of function develops but resolves when the blood flow is restored. TIAs are caused by a temporary blockage of an artery by a passing blood clot or a temporary inadequacy of blood flow through a narrowed artery. These brief attacks indicate that something is wrong with the system and so they warn of the possibility of a stroke. The risk of developing a stroke is highest in the hours, days and weeks after a TIA. Individuals with TIAs should seek immediate medical care.

LIFESTYLE MODIFICATIONS

Smoking

In *The Emperor of All Maladies*, Siddhartha Mukherjee writes eloquently on the history of cigarette smoking, the scientific studies that established the association between smoking and lung cancer, and the politics involving giant tobacco companies and governments.

> It remains an astonishing, disturbing fact that in America—a nation where nearly every new drug is subjected to rigorous scrutiny as a potential carcinogen, and even the bare hint of a

substance's link to cancer ignites a firestorm of public hysteria and media anxiety—one of the most potent and common carcinogens known to humans can be freely bought and sold at every corner store for a few dollars.

An example that illustrates this point even closer to home is the story of Maggi noodles in India.

Nestlé's Maggi first arrived in India in 1983. Maggi Instant Noodles started off as a snack for children, then became popular among students and young professionals, and today it can be found even in the most remote locations of the country, such as Himalayan trekking spots. According to the World Instant Noodles Association, India consumed 5,340 million cups or bags of instant noodles through 2014. Maggi was estimated to have a 70 per cent share of the market and contributed nearly 30 per cent to Nestlé's annual turnover.

However, in June 2015, Maggi, India's favourite two-minute snack, was pulled from the shelves after the Food Safety and Standards Authority of India (FSSAI) imposed a ban. It was labelled as 'unsafe and hazardous' for consumption. The ban was a result of experiments that found that the instant noodles contained huge quantities of taste enhancer monosodium glutamate (MSG) and lead, far beyond the permissible limit. The ban was imposed pan-India, and Nestlé was ordered not only to take Maggi off the shelves but also to destroy about 30,000 tonnes-worth of instant noodles, valued at nearly Rs 320 crore. A cement company was paid Rs 20 crore by Nestlé to burn the entire stock. A fine of about Rs 640 crore was levied on the company.

There was indeed a 'firestorm of public hysteria and media anxiety'. I was a medical student then and, like most other students in hostels across the country, was very fond of Maggi. It was a staple for many of us, and the news of its potential hazards was unsettling. We immediately discarded our stockpiles of Maggi and pondered over the damage it may have already done to us over the years.

Maggi returned to the shelves after being banned for about six months, armed this time with multiple clearances from government-certified laboratories.

Coming back to cigarettes, examining their components is alarming: there are approximately 600 ingredients in a cigarette. When burned, cigarettes produce more than 7,000 chemicals. About seventy of these chemicals are known to cause cancer, and many are toxic in other ways. Some of these chemicals are: acetone (found in nail polish remover), acetic acid (an ingredient in hair dye), ammonia (a common household cleaner), arsenic (used in rat poison), benzene (found in rubber, cement and gasoline), butane (used in lighter fluid), cadmium (an active component in battery acid), carbon monoxide (released in car exhaust fumes), formaldehyde (embalming fluid), hexamine (found in barbecue lighter fluid), lead (used in batteries), naphthalene (mothballs), methanol (rocket fuel), nicotine (insecticide), tar (material for paving roads) and toluene (used to make paint).

A definitive link has been established between smoking and cancers such as lung cancer, pancreatic cancer, bladder cancer, throat cancer, oesophageal cancer, kidney cancer and cervical cancer, to name a few. It causes a variety of lung diseases, such as chronic obstructive pulmonary disease, emphysema and chronic bronchitis. It also affects blood vessels throughout the body and causes Buerger's disease in the blood vessels of the arms and legs. Smoking causes aneurysms in the abdominal aorta. These aneurysms can rupture and can be rapidly fatal due to massive bleeding if not treated with emergency surgery.

Smoking increases the risk of haemorrhagic stroke as it causes hypertension. It also increases the tendency of formation of blood clots, which can lead to heart attacks and ischemic strokes. The more you smoke, the greater your risk of having a stroke. Smoke containing carbon monoxide and nicotine enters the bloodstream from the lungs. The carbon monoxide reduces the amount of oxygen in the blood, and the nicotine makes the heart beat faster and raises blood pressure. It can also trigger atrial fibrillation. Smoking reduces the level of good cholesterol, or HDL, and increases the level of bad cholesterol, or LDL.

Just as metal pipes carrying water rust over time and eventually burst and leak, smoking damages the blood vessels in the body over time. The chemicals from smoking travel in the blood and therefore they damage the blood vessels throughout the body, leading to their blockage or aneurysm formation in them. The bursting of an aneurysm is catastrophic.

In my opinion, people continue to smoke despite explicit warnings on cigarette packets because of two main reasons. Firstly, most people believe that smoking only causes lung cancer. Whenever I ask people to quit smoking, they often retort with anecdotes of people who have smoked for over forty or fifty years but haven't developed cancer. They are hopeful that they might be similarly lucky. The fact that lung cancer develops over a period of thirty years is the reason most people procrastinate quitting smoking till it becomes too late.

Secondly, even people who understand the health consequences of smoking and genuinely want to quit, can't. This is because of the addictive effect of nicotine. Nicotine causes a release of various neurotransmitters in the brain. One of them, dopamine, signals a pleasurable experience and is critical for reinforcing the effects of nicotine. Nicotine induces pleasure and reduces stress and anxiety. Smoking improves concentration, reaction time and certain task performances. This perceived enhancement is actually the abatement of withdrawal symptoms in smokers. Cessation of smoking causes withdrawal symptoms like irritability, depressed mood, restlessness and anxiety. The intensity of these mood disturbances is similar to that found in psychiatric patients. Anhedonia, the feeling that there is little pleasure in life, can also occur with withdrawal from nicotine.

Over the last twenty-five years, efforts geared towards smoking prevention and cessation, and public awareness campaigns describing the associated health risks regarding smoking, have enjoyed only limited success. What US Surgeon General C. Everett Koop said in 1982 still holds true: 'Cigarette smoking is clearly identified as the chief preventable cause of death in our society and the most important public health issue of our time.' Smoking greatly increases the risk of strokes in individuals who also have hypertension, diabetes or use oral contraceptive pills. Smokers who stop smoking have reduced risk of stroke and heart attacks than those who continue to smoke. The risk of stroke begins to revert about two years after quitting, and reverts to roughly that of a non-smoking person at the five-year mark.

Alcohol

The amount of alcohol that is consumed by an individual affects their stroke risk. Excessive alcohol intake increases the risk of brain haemorrhage. Light to moderate regular alcohol consumption appears to have a protective effect against carotid artery and systemic atherosclerosis, yet acute and chronic heavy use of alcohol increases ischemic stroke risk. The effect of alcohol as a risk factor is partially explained by the fact that individuals who consume large amounts of alcohol frequently have coexisting hypertension and are cigarette smokers. The exact type of alcohol consumed can play a role of its own, though the subject has not been well studied. Regular wine consumption confers a protective effect, beer and other spirits do not. The salutary effects of wine have been attributed to its non-alcoholic contents, especially to antioxidant flavonoids and tannins, which are believed to help guard against atherosclerosis. Grape juice might have the same effects as alcohol, although this remains a controversial hypothesis that has not been systematically studied.

Acute alcohol intoxication may precipitate ischemic strokes. Alcohol has a strong effect on the heart, which can further lead to strokes. It can damage the heart muscle and lead to alcoholic cardiomyopathy and can cause dysfunction in the heart rhythm, which is known as the holiday heart syndrome. These two can lead to ischemic stroke.

Alcoholic cardiomyopathy is defined as toxicity to the heart muscle by ethanol or its metabolites. Alcohol weakens the heart muscle and causes the heart to stretch and enlarge. The weakened heart muscle is unable to pump blood as effectively as it should.

Acute effects of alcohol can result in rhythm disturbances. Since this happens often on weekends and holidays when people binge drink, it is called the holiday heart syndrome. Ettinger and Regan coined the term and described thirty-two habitual drinkers who ingested an additional amount of ethanol prior to having an arrhythmia. Heavy drinkers have almost double the risk of atrial fibrillation as compared to non-drinkers. Atrial fibrillation can lead to clot formation, which can travel to the brain and cause ischemic stroke.

Migraines

I have myself been a sufferer of migraine headaches, which I experienced most frequently while in medical school. They were most common when I had to study for competitive exams, had overnight calls in the hospital or skipped meals. During an attack, I would just want to sleep in a dark room, away from any light or sound. Usually in most individuals, migraines are one sided. Some individuals may also get auras, such as flashing lights or zigzag lines in their field of vision, prior to an attack.

My headaches did have one positive side effect: they led to my first research project during my third year of medical school. I had become addicted to the popular mobile game Candy Crush Saga, but owing to my low threshold for headaches, I stopped playing altogether. Observing my colleagues play games on their phones for hours at a stretch and often till late at night, I thought it may be worthwhile to measure the magnitude of this potential gaming problem. I found that internet gaming disorder (IGD) was proposed as a 'condition for further study' by the Diagnostic and Statistical Manual of Mental Disorders, Fifth Edition (DSM-5). I then designed and conducted an IGD study on medical and dental students. This was one of the first studies reporting the prevalence of IGD in India and its effects on sleep, headache and cognition in young adults. We found that individuals with internet gaming disorder were more likely to develop headaches after prolonged gaming and that refraining from these games prevented headaches in them. We also found that individuals with IGD had poorer sleep quality and increased daytime drowsiness. They also had more nightmares due to violent games. Another intriguing correlation emerged between IGD and adult attention deficit hyperactivity disorder (ADHD).

Migraine is a hereditary condition that most often begins in early life and is more frequent in girls and women than in boys and men. During a migraine attack, arteries can narrow considerably, causing dizziness, disturbed vision, abnormal sensations like tingling and numbness and other neurologic symptoms. Conversely, migraines can also arise when arteries dilate, as this widening presses on the nerve endings on the outside of the arteries. This causes a headache, usually on just one side of the head. Vomiting and decreased fluid intake are common during a migraine attack. The dehydration and increased clotting tendency can lead to clots forming in the already narrowed arteries, leading to the development of a migrainous stroke in the portion of the brain supplied by the blocked artery. It is therefore advised to hydrate adequately during a migraine. Various medicines are available to either alleviate symptoms during a migraine attack or to prevent migraine attacks.

The presence of other stroke risk factors, such as hypertension, smoking and oral contraceptive use, compound the risk of stroke in patients with migraine.

15

World History and Stroke

This is a war to end all wars.

—Woodrow Wilson

Let us return, however, to the League of Nations. To create an organization which is in a position to protect peace in this world of conflicting interests and egoistic wills is a frighteningly difficult task.

—Hjalmar Branting

STROKE AND WORLD POLITICS

WOODROW WILSON, THE American president, envisioned the League of Nations as an instrument of peace—an international organization tasked with settling disputes without bloodshed. In January 1919, at the Paris Peace Conference that ended World War I, President Wilson persuaded the leaders from France, Great Britain and Italy to come together with the leaders of other nations to draft the Covenant of the League of Nations. While his idea got international support, it was vehemently opposed by the US Congress.

To garner support for the League, Wilson embarked on a very strenuous national tour on 22 August 1919, against the strong advice of his physician, Dr Grayson. Wilson was to cover 8,000 miles in twenty-two days and give two to three speeches every day. The gruelling tour schedule would take a serious toll on his health.

Previously, in 1906, at the age of fifty, Wilson woke up one morning blind in his left eye. The diagnosis suggested a left ophthalmic artery occlusion, possibly from an underlying left carotid artery disease. The attack was transient and his vision gradually improved.

As the tour took off in 1919, the president began experiencing severe headaches, which increased in both duration and intensity until he became almost blind during the attacks. As the tour neared its end, his headaches became even more debilitating, and he grew unusually restless. Suddenly, he developed a weakness on the left side of his face. Due to the gravity of the situation, the tour was cut short and Wilson began his journey back to Washington, DC. He suffered a complete stroke a week later. As described by his second wife, Edith Wilson:

> At 11, on Sunday morning, September 28, 1919, the train pulled its heavy way into Washington ... All the rest of the day my husband wandered like a ghost between the study at one end of the hall and my room at the other. The awful pain in his head that drove him relentlessly back and forth was too acute to permit work or even reading ... The next

day, the third since our return, the President seemed a little better. I had been sleeping fitfully, getting up every hour or so to see how my husband was ... At 5 or 6 in the morning, I found him sleeping normally, as it appeared. Relieved, I dozed off again until after 8. This time I found him sitting on the side of the bed trying to reach a water bottle. As I handed it to him, I noticed that his left hand hung loosely. 'I have no feeling in that hand,' he said. 'Will you rub it? But first help me to the bathroom.' He moved with great difficulty, and every move brought spasms of pain; with my help he gained the bathroom. It was so alarming that I asked if I could leave him long enough to telephone the doctor. He said yes, and hurrying into my room, I reached Dr Grayson at his house. While on the phone, I heard a slight noise and rushing into my husband's apartment I found him on the bathroom floor unconscious.

The only treatment available at that time was rest. The president was to be released from his difficult presidential duties till he became better.

Although Wilson was severely affected by his stroke, his illness was concealed by Edith, who shielded him from the outside world. Every document had to go through her, and she decided what was important for the president. Essentially, she ran a bedside government that excluded even Wilson's staff, the cabinet and the Congress. Wilson, on the other hand, became very rigid and would not acquiesce or compromise on anything when it came to the League of Nations. Any alterations proposed by the Senate were shot down, and the treaty was ultimately rejected.

His personality changes could have been a result of his stroke, for the League was initially his idea but he himself ended up driving it into the ground. The League of Nations was eventually formed without the United States as a member. While it met with some successes, it could not prevent World War II.

The history of the world has undoubtedly been altered by stroke, impacting the lives and careers of many world leaders. Both Vladimir Lenin and Woodrow Wilson, influential figures of the early twentieth century, experienced cognitive impairment owing to strokes they had while they were at helm of their countries at critical times in history. Lenin, at the age of fifty-two, suddenly developed dysarthria (difficulty speaking) and right hemiparesis. An observer noted that 'often as he spoke, the words were slurred and he paused several times like a man who had lost the thread of his argument'. The health status of political leaders is often concealed, especially when the illness is perceived as stigmatizing. It is no doubt that people would worry at the thought of having brought and left in power a cognitively impaired leader.

At the Yalta Conference, held from 4–11 February 1945, President Franklin D. Roosevelt of the United States, Soviet Union Premier Joseph Stalin and British Prime Minister Winston Churchill met to discuss how post-World War II Europe should be organized. All three men died within the next two decades of the conference. President Roosevelt died two months after the Yalta Conference due to a haemorrhagic stroke. Premier Stalin died eight years later, also due to a haemorrhagic stroke. Finally, Prime Minister Churchill died twenty years after the conference because of complications of stroke. The subsequent deterioration of these three leaders of the most powerful countries of the world had varying degrees of historical significance. Churchill's resignation following his illness led to Britain's mismanagement of the Egyptian Suez crisis and a period of mistrust with the United States. Roosevelt was still president and Stalin still premier at their times of passing, so their deaths carried huge political ramifications. The early death of Roosevelt may have exacerbated the post-World War II miscommunication between America and the Soviet Union, which may have precipitated the Cold War.

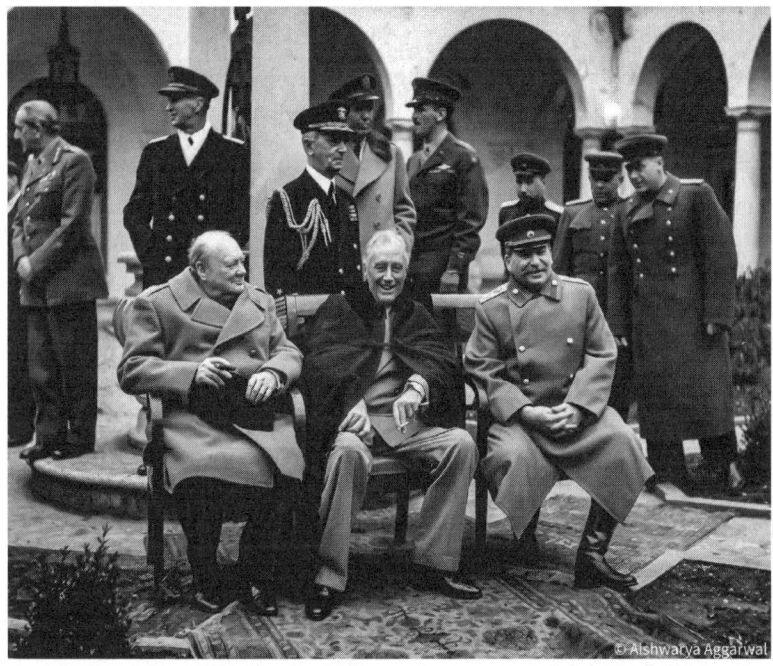

Figure 7 From left, Prime Minister Churchill, President Roosevelt and Premier Stalin at the 1945 Yalta Conference.

In a study titled 'Stroke and the American Presidency', the authors J. Meschia and B.E. Safirstein identified eight American presidents who suffered from stroke since 1846: John Quincy Adams, John Tyler, Millard Fillmore, Andrew Johnson, Chester

Arthur, Woodrow Wilson, Franklin D. Roosevelt and Richard M. Nixon. Of them, only John Tyler survived longer than a month following his last stroke. It's worth noting that some of the presidents who suffered strokes led unhealthy lifestyles. Chester Arthur was obese and got little exercise. Roosevelt was a heavy smoker and had severe uncontrolled hypertension. Andrew Johnson may have abused alcohol. Nixon represents the first president to be on scientifically validated preventive treatment—warfarin. He was also the first president to be considered for a controlled therapeutic trial in acute stroke and the first to have had an advanced directive regarding terminal care. President Dwight D. Eisenhower also suffered nonfatal strokes while in office. He made arrangements with Vice President Nixon on what would happen if he could not perform his duties as president. This idea became the basis of the 25th Amendment: 'In case of the removal of the President from office or of his death or resignation, the Vice President shall become President.' In a separate incident in 2000, former American president Gerald Ford exhibited signs of a stroke when he began slurring his words during a TV interview.

Many other popular historical figures including world leaders, musicians, artists, authors, pioneers in medicine and scientists, suffered strokes during their lives. Some of them are highlighted below.

WORLD LEADERS

Margaret Thatcher, the first female British prime minister, often referred to as the 'Iron Lady', died of a stroke on 8 April 2013.

Yasser Arafat, leader of the Palestine Liberation Organization and a recipient of the 1994 Nobel Peace Prize for his efforts towards establishing peace with Israeli leaders, died of a massive haemorrhage on 11 November 2004.

John A. Macdonald, the first prime minister of Canada, died of a stroke on 6 June 1891.

Alexander Mackenzie, the second prime minister of Canada, also died of a stroke on 17 April 1892.

Catherine the Great, the most renowned and the longest-ruling female leader of Russia, reigning from 1762 until 1796, marking a period known as Russia's Golden Age, died of a stroke on 6 November 1796.

Isambard Kingdom Brunel, one of the most famous figures of the British Industrial Revolution, died of a stroke on 15 September 1859.

Samuel de Champlain, the French explorer known for founding New France and Quebec City, died of a stroke on 25 December 1635.

Shirley Chisholm, the first Black Congresswoman in the United States, died of a stroke on 1 January 2005.

Ariel Sharon, the prime minister of Israel, was left in a prolonged state of unconsciousness after a series of strokes.

Atal Bihari Vajpayee, prime minister of India, suffered a stroke in 2009 that impaired his speech.

SCIENTISTS AND INVENTORS

Alexander von Humboldt, a naturalist and explorer whose quantitative work on botanical geography laid the foundation for the field of biogeography, died of a stroke on 6 May 1859.

John Logie Baird, the Scottish inventor of the television, died of a stroke on 14 June 1946.

Dorothy Hodgkin is best known for developing the crystallography of biochemical compounds. Her work in the determination of the molecular structure of penicillin and vitamin B12 earned her the 1964 Nobel Prize for Chemistry. She died of a stroke on 29 July 1994.

Henry Ford, the American industrialist and business magnate, founder of the Ford Motor Company and chief developer of the assembly line technique of mass production, died of a cerebral haemorrhage on 7 April 1947.

PIONEERS IN MEDICINE

William Harvey, the anatomist and physiologist who discovered blood circulation, died of a cerebral haemorrhage at the age of seventy-nine on 3 June 1657.

Marcello Malpighi, the discoverer of capillaries and the microscopic anatomy of the lungs, kidneys and spleen, died of an apoplectic right hemiplegia on 29 November 1694.

Edward Jenner, dubbed the 'father of immunology' and the inventor of the smallpox vaccine, died of a stroke on 26 January 1823. His work is said to have saved more lives than the work of any other human.

Louis Pasteur, known for his discoveries of the principles of vaccination, microbial fermentation and pasteurization, suffered a stroke at the age of forty-six, leading to left hemiparesis.

He rehabilitated himself and many of his greatest scientific achievements came after his stroke. After suffering multiple debilitating strokes, he died at the age of seventy-two on 28 September 1895.

Elizabeth Blackwell, the first woman to receive a medical degree in the United States and also the first woman on the UK medical register, died of a stroke on 31 May 1910.

Daniel Williams was an American heart surgeon who performed one of the first successful open-heart surgeries in the United States. He also founded the Provident Hospital in Chicago, the first African American-owned and operated hospital in America. He died of a stroke on 4 August 1931.

Three pivotal figures in twentieth-century neurology—Russell DeJong, the first editor of the journal *Neurology*; Raymond Escourolle, the French neuropathologist; and H. Houston Merritt, long time Columbia professor, writer of *Merritt's Neurology* and co-developer of the antiepileptic drug phenytoin—were severely disabled by multiple strokes in their later years.

Jill Bolte Taylor, an American neuroanatomist, author and international public speaker, experienced a massive cerebral haemorrhage following the rupture of an arterio-venous malformation in 1996, at the age of thirty-seven. Her subsequent eight-year recovery influenced her work as a scientist and speaker. It is the subject of her 2006 book *My Stroke of Insight: A Brain Scientist's Personal Journey*. Her TED talk on the subject was one of the first to go viral online, after which her book become a *New York Times* bestseller and was published in thirty languages.

AUTHORS

Charles Dickens, regarded as the greatest novelist of the Victorian era, died of a stroke at the age of fifty-eight on 9 June 1870.

Anne Morrow Lindbergh, an acclaimed author and the first licensed female glider pilot in the United States, died of a stroke at the age of ninety-four on 7 February 2001.

Bram Stoker, the Irish author of the 1897 Gothic novel *Dracula*, died of a stroke on 20 April 1912.

Louisa May Alcott, the author of the acclaimed titles *Little Women*, *Little Men* and *Jo's Boys*, died from a stroke at the age of fifty-five on 6 March 1888.

Edith Wharton, the Pulitzer Prize laureate, died of a stroke on 11 August 1937.

ACTORS AND MUSICIANS

Charlie Chaplin, the British comedian, actor and filmmaker, died of a stroke at the age of eighty-eight on 25 December 1977.

Grace Kelly, a Golden Globe- and Oscar-winning actress died following a crash resulting from a stroke on 14 September 1982.

Luke Perry, an American actor most known for his role in the teenage drama *Beverly Hills, 90210*, died of a stroke on 4 March 2019.

Game of Thrones star Emilia Clarke suffered complications from her brain aneurysms in 2011 and 2013 (discussed in Chapter 9).

Johann Sebastian Bach, celebrated for his exceptional compositions during the Baroque period, died of a stroke on 28 July 1750.

Felix Mendelssohn, the German composer and pianist who was central to the Romantic era, died of a stroke on 4 November 1847.

Giuseppe Verdi, a dominant Italian composer of the nineteenth century, recognized for his unique style of opera, died of a stroke on 27 January 1901.

Sergei Prokofiev, a prolific Russian composer, pianist and conductor regarded as one of the most influential composers of the twentieth century, died of a cerebral haemorrhage at the age of sixty-one on 5 March 1953. This day coincided with Joseph Stalin's death. Prokofiev had lived near Red Square, and for three days, throngs of people gathered to mourn Stalin, making it impossible to hold Prokofiev's funeral at the headquarters of the Soviet Composers' Union. His coffin had to be moved by hand through the back streets, away from the vast crowds paying homage to Stalin.

Acknowledgements

I CONCEIVED THE idea of this book five years ago while studying for my final year medical school exams. It's funny how the brain gets distracted during exam time and drifts to the most creative ideas. This never seems to happen when you're actually free—only when you're supposed to focus on something else. As soon as my final exams were behind me, I started to look for material for this book. I wanted to explore the complexities of stroke and its far-reaching impact. The following year, which is the internship year, is typically very hectic. It is also when people start to prepare for competitive exams to get into a post-graduation course. But I felt so strongly about this book that I kept at it. My research for the book and my clinical training complemented each other. I would observe various clinical procedures, which stimulated my reading, and my wide research for the book led to better observations while in the hospital.

Since those early days, I have gained invaluable experience caring for patients. It is both humbling and rewarding to witness the transformative impact of timely interventions, and these experiences have only deepened my commitment to advancing stroke care.

My vision for the future is one where every patient, regardless of geography or circumstances, has access to life-saving treatments like thrombolysis and thrombectomy. Equally important is our collective effort to prevent strokes, through education, awareness and healthier living.

Writing this book has been a journey of discovery—not just about the history and science of stroke but also about the human stories behind it. I hope the book inspires readers to prioritize a healthy lifestyle and sparks conversations about the importance of accessible, equitable stroke care.

My father, Dr Anil Aggarwal, and my mother, Dr Saroj Aggarwal, have been pillars of inspiration. Throughout my childhood, I saw how demanding their professional lives were. Yet they never complained about their schedules. They were driven by purpose and passion, and they felt rewarded by the gratitude and respect offered by their patients. I grew up hearing stories about their patients and the impact of treatment, which inspired me to pursue medicine.

My mother has a huge collection of medical fiction and non-fiction books, and I started reading them at an early age. Almost all the accomplished writers I look up to, say that to write well you have to become a good reader first, and I owe my reading habit to my mother. Although my parents initially had concerns about my taking up writing a book instead of focusing on the competitive entrance tests, they were onboard after reading some of my initial work. In fact, my mother was the first reviewer of every chapter that I wrote.

I got into academic writing with my first paper on internet gaming disorder. My mentor for the paper, Dr Jeyaraj Pandian, the current president of the World Stroke Organization, appreciated my work and asked me to author a book chapter on haemorrhagic cerebrovascular diseases with him. I enjoyed the process of reviewing literature for my work on the paper and the chapter, and felt a strong need to write more. While reviewing the literature for the chapter, I came across various terms such as Charcot-Bouchard aneurysms and then delved into their origins. I am grateful to Dr Pandian for giving me that opportunity and for his consistent encouragement and feedback on some of these chapters, which served as an impetus for me to write more. I am also grateful to Dr Akanksha William at Christian Medical College (CMC) for her insights into various research methodologies.

It is because I was greatly inspired by Siddhartha Mukherjee's *The Emperor of All Maladies*, that I decided to write this book. And when I embarked on the project, the first book that I read on the subject of stroke was *Navigating the Complexities of Stroke* by Dr Louis R. Caplan. This book and another of his renowned texts, *Caplan's Stroke: A Clinical Approach*, served as my main reference sources. I take pride in the fact that I possess one of Dr Caplan's signed personal copies. When I first watched Dr Caplan's interview with Charles Miller Fisher, I was in awe of the two neurologists. Never in my wildest dreams could I have imagined that one day I would sit with Dr Caplan in his own office and work as his mentee. Dr Caplan and his vast body of work have guided me along this journey. He is a great clinician and academician, and I deeply treasure the clinical experience that I gained from him. I learnt from him the value of not only treating your patients but also teaching them how to lead better lives. Observing him escort his patients from the waiting area to the examination room, his detailed history-taking, and the nuances of his clinical examinations and personalization of care really inspired me. He often narrated his life experiences and anecdotes from his time with Miller Fisher, which were both entertaining and enlightening, and some of which I have included in this book. He taught me humility and kindness, and I aspire to be a clinician and an academician like him.

Many other texts have served as sources of inspiration and information for this book. Some of them are: *The Gene: An Intimate History; The Laws of Medicine: Field Notes from an Uncertain Science; Diabetes: The Biography; Brainstorm: Detective Stories from the World of Neurology; The Man Who Mistook His Wife for a Hat; Heart: A History; tPA for Stroke: The Story of a Controversial Drug; Visualizing Disease: The Art and History of Pathological Illustrations; The Greatest Benefit to Mankind: A Medical History of Humanity; Phantoms in the Brain: Probing the Mysteries of the Human Mind; Minds behind the Brain: A History of the Pioneers and their Discoveries; Medicine's 10 Greatest Discoveries; My Stroke of Insight: A Brain Scientist's Personal Journey; Being Mortal: Medicine and What Matters in the End; The Invention of Surgery: A History of Modern Medicine; Striking Back at Stroke: A Doctor–Patient Journal; The Brain that Changes Itself;* and *King of Hearts: The True Story of the Maverick Who Pioneered Open Heart Surgery.*

My understanding of the technicalities of writing and the publishing process also owes much to books like *On Writing Well* by William Zinsser; *Publishing Confidential* by Paul B. Brown; and *How to Get Published in India* by Meghna Pant.

I am grateful to Red Ink Literary Agency for representing my work. Many thanks to the wonderful team of editors and designers at HarperCollins for their efforts. Special thanks to Udayan Mitra, Gayatri Goswami and Janaki Sundaram at HarperCollins.

To everyone who has supported me and guided me along this journey, I offer my deepest gratitude. And to you, the reader, thank you for joining me in this effort to make a meaningful difference in stroke care. Together, we can strive for a future where the burden of stroke is significantly diminished and where lives are saved every day.

References

INTRODUCTION

1. Engelhardt E. Apoplexy, cerebrovascular disease, and stroke: Historical evolution of terms and definitions. Dement Neuropsychol. 2017; 11(4): 449–53.
2. Humorism. In: Wikipedia [Internet]. 2021 [cited 2021 Apr 11]. Available from: https://en.wikipedia.org/w/index.php?title=Humorism&oldid=1016738777.
3. Coupland AP, Thapar A, Qureshi MI, Jenkins H, Davies AH. The definition of stroke. J R Soc Med. 2017 Jan 1; 110(1): 9–12.
4. Schiller F. Concepts of stroke before and after Virchow. Med Hist. 1970 Apr; 14(2): 115–31.
5. Learn about stroke. In: World Stroke Organization [Internet]. [cited 2021 Apr 11]. Available from: https://www.world-stroke.org/world-stroke-day-campaign/why-stroke-matters/learn-about-stroke.

6. Caplan LR. Navigating the Complexities of Stroke. (Brain and Life Books). Oxford, New York: Oxford University Press; 2013. 288 p.
7. Saver JL. Time Is Brain—Quantified. Stroke. 2006 Jan 1; 37(1): 263–66.

1. THE CIRCLE OF WILLIS

1. Caplan LR, Aggarwal A. Andreas Vesalius. In: Stories of Stroke: Key Individuals and the Evolution of Ideas. Cambridge: Cambridge University Press; 2022. 21–24
2. Lo WB, Ellis H. The circle before Willis: a historical account of the intracranial anastomosis. Neurosurgery. 2010 Jan; 66(1): 7–18; discussion 17–18.
3. O'Connor JPB. Thomas Willis and the background to Cerebri Anatome. J R Soc Med. 2003 Mar; 96(3): 139–43.
4. The Invisible College (1645–1658). [Internet]. [cited 2018 Jul 31]. Available from: https://technicaleducationmatters.org/2010/12/12/the-invisible-college-1645-1658/.
5. Pearce JMS. Historical Note on Carotid Disease and Ligation. Eur Neurol. 2014; 72(1–2): 26–29.
6. Porter R. The Greatest Benefit to Mankind: A Medical History of Humanity from Antiquity to the Present. London: HarperCollins; 1997. 882 p.
7. Brenner E. Human body preservation—old and new techniques. J Anat. 2014 Mar; 224(3): 316–44.
8. Embalming. In: Wikipedia [Internet]. 2021 [cited 2021 Apr 11]. Available from: https://en.wikipedia.org/w/index.php?title=Embalming&oldid=1014790326.

9. Meli DB. Visualizing Disease: The Art and History of Pathological Illustrations. Chicago: University of Chicago Press; 2018. 311 p.
10. Lithography. In: Wikipedia [Internet]. 2020 [cited 2020 Aug 22]. Available from: https://en.wikipedia.org/w/index.php?title=Lithography&oldid=972927973.
11. Lithography. In: Encyclopaedia Britannica [Internet]. [cited 2020 Aug 22]. Available from: https://www.britannica.com/technology/lithography.
12. Munster AB, Thapar A, Davies AH. History of Carotid Stroke. Stroke. 2016 Apr; 47(4): e66-69. DOI: 10.1161/STROKEAHA.115.012044. Epub 2016 Jan 21. PMID: 26797663.

2. ON THE MOTION OF THE HEART AND BLOOD

1. Friedman M, Friedland GW. Medicine's 10 Greatest Discoveries. New Haven: Yale University Press; 2000.
2. Porter R. The Greatest Benefit to Mankind: A Medical History of Humanity from Antiquity to the Present. London: HarperCollins; 1997. 882 p.
3. Royal College of Physicians. How William Harvey discovered the circulation of the blood and why he regretted it. In: Youtube [Internet]. [cited 2018 Sep 8]. Available from: https://www.youtube.com/watch?v=ZR8LmpfkXhQ
4. A giant leap for mankind: William Harvey reveals the circulation of the blood. In: History Extra [Internet]. [cited 2018 Aug 12]. Available from: https://www.historyextra.com/period/stuart/william-harvey-reveals-the-circulation-of-the-blood/.

5. Ribatti D. William Harvey and the discovery of the circulation of the blood. J Angiogenesis Res. 2009 Sep 21; 1: 3.
6. ME Silverman. William Harvey and the Discovery of the Circulation of Blood. Clinical Cardiology. 1985; 8: 244–26. In: Wiley Online Library [Internet]. [cited 2018 Sep 9]. Available from: https://onlinelibrary.wiley.com/doi/abs/10.1002/clc.4960080411.
7. Andrioli G, Trincia G. Padua. The renaissance of human anatomy and medicine. Neurosurgery. 2004 Oct; 55(4): 746–54; discussion 755.
8. Bloodletting and blisters: Solving the medical mystery of George Washington's death. In: PBS NewsHour [Internet]. 2014 [cited 2018 Sep 5]. Available from: https://www.pbs.org/newshour/show/bloodletting-blisters-solving-medical-mystery-george-washingtons-death.
9. The history of bloodletting. In: BC-Medical Journal [Internet]. [cited 2018 Aug 22]. Available from: https://www.bcmj.org/premise/history-bloodletting.
10. Parapia LA. History of bloodletting by phlebotomy. Br J Haematol. 2008 Nov 1; 143(4): 490–95.
11. Dissections banned in Indian universities. In: Science. AAAS [Internet]. [cited 2021 Apr 29]. Available from: https://www.sciencemag.org/news/2014/08/dissections-banned-indian-universities.
12. Local blood flow regulation. In: Wikipedia [Internet]. 2020 [cited 2021 Apr 29]. Available from: https://en.wikipedia.org/w/index.php?title=Local_blood_flow_regulation&oldid=934807313.
13. Roy CS, Sherrington CS. On the Regulation of the Blood-supply of the Brain. J Physiol. 1890 Jan; 11(1-2): 85–158.17.

14. Fulton JF. Observations upon the Vascularity of the Human Occipital Lobe during Visual Activity. Brain. 1928 Oct 1; 51(3): 310–20.
15. Caplan L, Liebeskind D. Pathology, anatomy, and pathophysiology of stroke. In: Caplan L, editor. Caplan's Stroke: A Clinical Approach. Cambridge: Cambridge University Press; 2016. 19–54.

3. VIRCHOW'S TRIAD

1. History of pathology. In: Wikipedia [Internet]. 2021 [cited 2021 May 5]. Available from: https://en.wikipedia.org/w/index.php?title=History_of_pathology&oldid=1002588983.
2. Meli DB. Visualizing Disease: The Art and History of Pathological Illustrations. Chicago: University of Chicago Press; 2018. 311 p.
3. Walter E, Scott M. The life and work of Rudolf Virchow 1821–1902: 'Cell theory, thrombosis and the sausage duel.' J Intensive Care Soc. 2017 Aug; 18(3): 234–35.
4. Schultz M. Rudolf Virchow. Emerg Infect Dis. 2008 Sep; 14(9): 1480–81.
5. Bagot CN, Arya R. Virchow and his triad: A question of attribution. Br J Haematol. 2008 Sep 24; 143(2): 180–90.
6. Kumar DR, Hanlin E, Glurich I, Mazza JJ, Yale SH. Virchow's Contribution to the Understanding of Thrombosis and Cellular Biology. Clin Med Res. 2010 Dec; 8(3–4): 168–72.
7. Schiller F. Concepts of stroke before and after Virchow. Med Hist. 1970 Apr; 14(2): 115–31.
8. Ackerknecht EH. Rudolf Virchow: Doctor, Statesman, Anthropologist. Madison (WI): University of Wisconsin; 1953.

9. Storey CE, Pols H. Chapter 27: A History of Cerebrovascular Disease. Handb Clin Neurol. 2010; 95: 401–15.
10. Maurizio Paciaroni, Julien Bogousslavsky. Chapter 1: The history of stroke and cerebrovascular disease. Handb of Clin Neurol. 2008; 92: 3–28.
11. Safavi-Abbasi S, Reis C, Talley MC, Theodore N, Nakaji P, Spetzler RF, et al. Rudolf Ludwig Karl Virchow: Pathologist, physician, anthropologist, and politician. Implications of his work for the understanding of cerebrovascular pathology and stroke. Neurosurg Focus. 2006 Jun 15; 20(6): E1.

4. THE HEART AND BRAIN CONNECTION

1. Storey CE, Pols H. Chapter 27: A History of Cerebrovascular Disease. Handb Clin Neurol. 2010; 95: 401–15.
2. The Death of President Franklin Roosevelt, 1945. [Internet]. [cited 2019 Feb 27]. Available from: http://www.eyewitnesstohistory.com/fdrdeath.htm.
3. Harold on History. In: Historical Perspectives on Hypertension [Internet]. American College of Cardiology. [cited 2019 Feb 27]. Available from: https://www.acc.org/latest-in-cardiology/articles/2017/11/14/14/42/harold-on-history-historical-perspectives-on-hypertension.
4. History of hypertension. In: Wikipedia [Internet]. 2019 [cited 2019 Feb 27]. Available from: https://en.wikipedia.org/w/index.php?title=History_of_hypertension&oldid=883568076.
5. Kumar V, Abbas AK, Aster JC. Robbins Basic Pathology. Elsevier Health Sciences; 2013. 925 p.
6. Chopra HK, Nanda NC. Textbook of Cardiology: A Clinical and Historical Perspective. Jaypee Brothers Medical Publishers Pvt. Ltd.; 2013. 805 p.

7. AlGhatrif M, Lindsay J. A brief review: History to understand fundamentals of electrocardiography. J Community Hosp Intern Med Perspect. 2012 Apr 30; 2(1).
8. Mehta NJ, Khan IA. Cardiology's 10 greatest discoveries of the 20th century. Tex Heart Inst J. 2002; 29(3): 164–71.
9. Barold SS. Willem Einthoven and the birth of clinical electrocardiography a hundred years ago. Card Electrophysiol Rev. 2003 Jan; 7(1): 99–104.
10. Edler I, Lindström K. The history of echocardiography. Ultrasound Med Biol. 2004 Dec; 30(12): 1565–644.
11. Feigenbaum H. Evolution of Echocardiography. Circulation 1996; 93: 1321–327.
12. Edler I, Gustafson A, Karlefors T, Christensson B. Ultrasound cardiography. Acta Med Scand Suppl. 1961; 370: 5–123.
13. Framingham Heart Study. In: Wikipedia [Internet]. 2021 [cited 2021 May 17]. Available from: https://en.wikipedia.org/w/index.php?title=Framingham_Heart_Study&oldid=1020777199.
14. Atherosclerosis. In: Wikipedia [Internet]. 2021 [cited 2021 May 21]. Available from: https://en.wikipedia.org/w/index.php?title=Atherosclerosis&oldid=1022543037.
15. Nassief A, Marsh JD. Statin therapy for stroke prevention. Stroke. 2008 Mar; 39(3): 1042–48.

5. NO-MAN'S LAND

1. AANS Neurosurgery. C. Miller Fisher, MD interviewed by Louis R. Caplan, MD [Internet]. [cited 2018 Jul 19]. Available from: https://www.youtube.com/watch?v=A6krI_HUyPs.
2. Caplan LR, Mohr JP, Ackerman RH. In Memoriam: Charles Miller Fisher, MD (1913–2012). *Arch Neurol.* 2012; 69(9): 1208–209.

3. Estol CJ. Dr C. Miller Fisher and the History of Carotid Artery Disease. Stroke. 1996 Mar 1; 27(3): 559–66.
4. Munster AB, Thapar A, Davies AH. History of Carotid Stroke. Stroke. 2016 Apr 1; 47(4): e66–69.
5. Pearce JMS. Historical Note on Carotid Disease and Ligation. Eur Neurol. 2014; 72(1–2): 26–29.
6. Robicsek F, Roush TS, Cook JW, Reames MK. From Hippocrates to Palmaz-Schatz, The History of Carotid Surgery. Eur J Vasc Endovasc Surg. 2004 Apr 1; 27(4): 389–97.
7. T Robertson J. Carotid Endarterectomy: A Saga of Clinical Science, Personalities, and Evolving Technology: The Willis Lecture. Stroke. 1998 Dec 1; 29: 2435–441.
8. DeBakey ME. Successful Carotid Endarterectomy For Cerebrovascular Insufficiency: Nineteen-Year Follow-up. JAMA. 1975 Sep 8; 233(10): 1083–085.
9. Easton JD. History of Carotid Endarterectomy Then and Now: Personal Perspective. Stroke. 2014 Jun 1; 45(6): e101–03.
10. Thompson JE. The Evolution of Surgery for the Treatment and Prevention of Stroke: The Willis Lecture. Stroke. 1996 Aug 1; 27(8): 1427–434.
11. Menzoian JO. On the 60th anniversary of carotid surgery for the prevention of stroke. J Vasc Surg. 2014 May; 59(5): 1465–468.
12. Fisher CM. Occlusion of the Internal Carotid Artery. Arch Neurol Psychiatry. 1951 Mar 1; 65(3): 346–77.
13. Tallarita T, Gerbino M, Gurrieri C, Lanzino G. History of carotid surgery: From ancient Greeks to the modern era. Perspect Vasc Surg Endovasc Ther. 2013 Dec; 25(3–4): 57–64.
14. Thompson JE. The Development of Carotid Artery Surgery. Arch Surg. 1973 Nov 1; 107(5): 643–48.

15. Friedman SG. The first carotid endarterectomy. J Vasc Surg. 2014 Dec; 60(6): 1703–708. e1–4.
16. Cooper, A. Account of the first successful operation performed on the common carotid artery for aneurysm in the year 1808, with post-mortem examination in 1821. Guy's Hosp. Rep. 1836; 1: 53–59.

6. BLOOD THINNERS

1. Couch NP. About heparin, or ... whatever happened to Jay McLean? J Vasc Surg. 1989 Jul; 10(1): 1–8.
2. Marcum JA. Discovery of Heparin: Contributions of William Henry Howell and Jay McLean. Physiology. 1992 Oct; 7(5): 237–42.
3. Mclean J. The Discovery of Heparin. Circulation. 1959 Jan; 19(1): 75–78.
4. McLean J. The Thromboplastic Action of Cephalin. Am J Physiol. 1916 Aug 1; 41(2): 250–57.
5. Charles AF, Scott DA. Studies on Heparin: I. the Preparation of Heparin. J Biol Chem. 1933 Oct 1; 102(2): 425–29.
6. Lever, R, Mulloy, B and Page, C. Heparin—A Century Of Progress. Alemania: Springer Healthcare Ltd; 2012. pp. 4–18.
7. Oduah EI, Linhardt RJ, Sharfstein ST. Heparin: Past, Present, and Future. Pharmaceuticals (Basel) 2016 Jul 4; 9(3): 38.
8. Caplan L, Saver J. Treatment. In: Caplan L, editor. Caplan's Stroke: A Clinical Approach. Cambridge: Cambridge University Press; 2016. 170–77.
9. Saxena R, Lewis S, Berge E, Sandercock PA, Koudstaal PJ. Risk of early death and recurrent stroke and effects of heparin in

3169 patients with acute ischemic stroke and atrial fibrillation in the International Stroke Trial. Stroke. 2001; 32: 2333–337.
10. Resnick SB, Resnick SH, Weintraub JL, Kothary N. Heparin in Interventional Radiology: A Therapy in Evolution. Semin Interv Radiol. 2005 Jun; 22(2): 95–107.
11. Link KP. The Discovery of Dicumarol and Its Sequels. Circulation. 1959 Jan 1; 19(1): 97–107.
12. Wardrop D, Keeling D. The story of the discovery of heparin and warfarin. Br J Haematol. 2008 Jun 1; 141(6): 757–63.
13. Biographical Memoirs: V.65. In: Nat Acad Press [Internet]. [cited 2018 Feb 18]. Available from: https://www.nap.edu/read/4548/chapter/9.
14. This month in 1939: How dead cattle led to the discovery of warfarin. In: PMLive [Internet]. 2013 [cited 2018 Feb 3]. Available from: http://www.pmlive.com/pharma_news/how_dead_cattle_led_to_the_discovery_of_warfarin_485464.
15. Doctrine of signatures. In: Brought to Life [Internet]. [cited 2018 Apr 15]. Available from: http://broughttolife.sciencemuseum.org.uk/broughttolife/techniques/doctrine.
16. A history of aspirin. In: Pharmaceutical Journal [Internet]. [cited 2018 Apr 12]. Available from: https://www.pharmaceutical-journal.com/news-and-analysis/infographics/a-history-of-aspirin/20066661.article.
17. Stone E. XXXII. An account of the success of the bark of the willow in the cure of agues. In a letter to the Right Honourable George Earl of Macclesfield, President of R. S. from the Rev. Mr. Edward Stone, of Chipping-Norton in Oxfordshire. Philos Trans. 1763 Jan 1; 53: 195–200.
18. Jack DB. One hundred years of aspirin. The Lancet. 1997 Aug 9; 350(9075): 437–39.

19. The Controversial Story of Aspirin. In: World Neurology Online [Internet]. [cited 2018 Apr 9]. Available from: https://worldneurologyonline.com/article/controversial-story-aspirin/.
20. Buchanan WW, Kean WF. The treatment of acute rheumatism by salicin, by T.J. Maclagan—The Lancet, 1876. J Rheumatol. 2002 Jun 1; 29(6): 1321–323.
21. Snead MW, Aikawa JK. T.J. Maclagan and the Treatment of Rheumatic Fever with Salicin. AMA Arch Intern Med. 1958 May 1; 101(5): 997–1004.
22. Jesus Malverde. How aspirin turned hero - Heroin, Bayer and Heinrich Dreser. In: Democratic Underground [Internet]. [cited 2018 Apr 12]. Available from: https://www.democraticunderground.com/11701737.
23. Lichterman BL. Aspirin: The Story of a Wonder Drug. BMJ. 2004 Dec 11; 329(7479): 1408.
24. Miner J, Hoffhines A. The Discovery of Aspirin's Antithrombotic Effects. Tex Heart Inst J. 2007; 34(2): 179–86.

7. CLOT BUSTERS AND RETRIEVERS

1. Busch C. The Serendipity Mindset: The Art and Science of Creating Good Luck. New York: Riverhead Books; 2020.
2. Gray D. Thrombolysis: past, present, and future. Postgrad Med J. 2006 Jun; 82(968): 372–75.
3. The rise and fall of the clot buster: A review on the history of Streptokinase. (2014). In The Pharmaceutical Journal [Internet]. Available from: https://doi.org/10.1211/PJ.2014.20065679.
4. Sherry S. The origin of thrombolytic therapy. J Am Coll Cardiol. 1989 Oct 1; 14(4): 1085–92.

5. Mueller RL, Scheidt S. History of drugs for thrombotic disease. Discovery, development, and directions for the future. Circulation. 1994 Jan; 89(1): 432–49.
6. Clot Busters! Discovery of Thrombolytic Therapy for Heart & Stroke. In: FASEB [Internet]. [cited 2018 Jul 19]. Available from: http://faseb.org/Resources-for-the-Public/News-Room/Article-Detail-View/tabid/1014/ArticleId/1260/Clot-Busters-Discovery-of-Thrombolytic-Therapy-for-Heart-Stroke.aspx.
7. Zivin JA, Simmons JG. tPA for Stroke: The Story of a Controversial Drug. Oxford: Oxford University Press; 2010. 206 p.
8. Collen D, Lijnen HR. Tissue-type plasminogen activator: A historical perspective and personal account. J Thromb Haemost. 2004 Apr; 2(4): 541–46.
9. Sikri N, Bardia A. A History of Streptokinase Use in Acute Myocardial Infarction. Tex Heart Inst J. 2007; 34(3): 318–27.
10. Maroo A, Topol EJ. The early history and development of thrombolysis in acute myocardial infarction. J Thromb Haemost. 2004 Nov; 2: 1867–70.
11. Caplan L, Saver, J. Treatment. In: Caplan L, editor. Caplan's Stroke: A Clinical Approach. Cambridge: Cambridge University Press; 2016. pp. 145–216.

8. IMAGING

1. Caplan LR. Navigating the Complexities of Stroke. (Brain and Life Books). Oxford, New York: Oxford University Press; 2013. 288 p.
2. Digital subtraction angiography. Radiology Reference Article. In: Radiopaedia.org [Internet]. [cited 2021 Apr 30]. Available

from: https://radiopaedia.org/articles/digital-subtraction-angiography.
3. Antunes JL. Egas Moniz and cerebral angiography. J Neurosurg. 1974 Apr 1; 40(4): 427–32.
4. Artico M, Spoletini M, Fumagalli L, Biagioni F, Ryskalin L, Fornai F, et al. Egas Moniz: 90 Years (1927–2017) from Cerebral Angiography. Front Neuroanat. 2017 Sep 1; 11: 81.
5. Doby T. Cerebral angiography and Egas Moniz. Am J Roentgenol. 1992 Aug 1; 159(2): 364.
6. Ferro JM. Egas Moniz and Internal Carotid Occlusion. Arch Neurol. 1988 May 1; 45(5): 563–64.
7. Ligon BL. The Mystery of Angiography and the "Unawarded" Nobel Prize: Egas Moniz and Hans Christian Jacobaeus. Neurosurgery. 1998 Sep 1; 43(3): 602–11.
8. Manoel Bertolote J. Egas Moniz: Twice a double life. Arq Neuropsiquiatr. 2015 Oct 1; 73: 885–86.
9. Duarte G, Goulão A. Editorial. Egas moniz, the pioneer of cerebral angiography. Interv Neuroradiol J Peritherapeutic Neuroradiol Surg Proced Relat Neurosci. 1997 Jun 30; 3(2): 107–11.
10. González-Crussi, F. A Short History of Medicine. New York: Modern Library, 2008.
11. Gajera J. Seldinger technique. Radiology Reference Article. In: Radiopaedia.org [Internet]. [cited 2021 Apr 30]. Available from: https://radiopaedia.org/articles/seldinger-technique?lang=us.
12. Seldinger technique. In: Wikipedia [Internet]. 2020 [cited 2021 Apr 30]. Available from: https://en.wikipedia.org/w/index.php?title=Seldinger_technique&oldid=984288047.
13. The Nobel Prize in Physiology or Medicine 1979. In: NobelPrize.org. [Internet]. [cited 2018 Oct 23]. Available from: https://www.nobelprize.org/prizes/medicine/1979/ceremony-speech/.

14. Doctor Klioze. History of Computerized Tomography (CT Scanner). In: Youtube [Internet]. [cited 2018 Oct 25]. Available from: https://www.youtube.com/watch?v=9SUHgtREWQc.
15. xrayctscanner. The Scanner Story (Part 1 of 2 of documentary covering early CT development). In: Youtube [Internet]. [cited 2018 Oct 29]. Available from: https://www.youtube.com/watch?v=u_R47LDdlZM.
16. Allan M. Cormack. Nobel Lecture: Early Two-Dimensional Reconstruction and Recent Topics Stemming from It. In: NobelPrize.org [Internet]. [cited 2020 Apr 20]. Available from: https://www.nobelprize.org/prizes/medicine/1979/cormack/lecture/.
17. The Beatles, the Nobel Prize, and CT scanning of the chest. In: PubMed NCBI [Internet]. [cited 2020 Apr 20]. Available from: https://www.ncbi.nlm.nih.gov/pubmed/19995626.
18. Godfrey N. Hounsfield. Nobel Lecture: Computed Medical Imaging. In: NobelPrize.org [Internet]. [cited 2020 Apr 20]. Available from: https://www.nobelprize.org/prizes/medicine/1979/hounsfield/lecture/.
19. Kinley, Jeff, and R Damadian. Gifted Mind: The Dr. Raymond Damadian Story, Inventor of the MRI. Master Books; 2015.
20. Dawson MJ. Paul Lauterbur and the Invention of MRI. Cambridge: MIT Press; 2013. 324 p.
21. Mansfield P. The Long Road to Stockholm: The Story of Magnetic Resonance Imaging– An Autobiography. Oxford: Oxford University Press, 2013.
22. Dreizen P. The Nobel prize for MRI: A wonderful discovery and a sad controversy. Lancet. 2004 Jan 3; 363(9402): 78.
23. Prize Fight. In: Smithsonian [Internet]. [cited 2019 Jun 10]. Available from: https://www.smithsonianmag.com/science-nature/prize-fight-95652491/.

24. Lauterbur PC. Magnetic resonance zeugmatography. *Pure and Applied Chemistry.* 1974; *40(1–2):* 149–57.
25. The Nobel Prize in Physiology or Medicine 2003. In: NobelPrize.org. [Internet]. [cited 2019 Jun 10]. Available from: https://www.nobelprize.org/prizes/medicine/2003/lauterbur/biographical/.
26. Macchia RJ, Termine JE, Buchen CD. Raymond V. Damadian, M.D.: Magnetic resonance imaging and the controversy of the 2003 Nobel Prize in Physiology or Medicine. J Urol. 2007 Sep; 178(3 Pt 1): 783–85.
27. Rich DA. A brief history of positron emission tomography. J Nucl Med Technol. 1997 Mar 1; 25(1): 4 –11.
28. Positron discovered. In: Physics Today [Internet]. August 2, 2016. [cited 2020 Apr 20] Available from: https://physicstoday.scitation.org/do/10.1063/PT.5.031277/abs/.
29. The Nobel Prize in Physics 1936. In: NobelPrize.org [Internet]. Available from: www.nobelprize.org/prizes/physics/1936/anderson/biographical/.
30. Rhodes R. The Making of the Atomic Bomb. New York: Simon and Schuster; 1995.
31. The Nobel Prize. Women who changed science: Irene Joliot-Curie. In: NobelPrize.org. [Internet]. [cited 2020 Apr 20] Available from: www.nobelprize.org/womenwhochangedscience/stories/irene-joliot-curie.
32. The Nobel Prize in Chemistry 1935. In: NobelPrize.org [Internet]. [cited 2020 Apr 20]. Available from: www.nobelprize.org/prizes/chemistry/1935/joliot-fred/biographical/.
33. Joliot F, Curie I. Artificial production of a new kind of radio-element. Nature. 1934 Feb 1; 133(3554): 201–02.
34. Wagner HN. A brief history of positron emission tomography (PET). Semin. Nucl. Med. 1998 Jul 1; 28(3): 213–20.

35. Bailey DL, Townsend DW, Valk PE, Maisey MN. Positron Emission Tomography: Basic Sciences. London: Springer-Verlag; 2005.
36. Portnow LH, Vaillancourt DE, Okum MS. The history of cerebral PET scanning. Neurology 2013 Mar 5; 80(10): 952–56.
37. Raichle ME. A brief history of human brain mapping. Trends Neurosci. 2009 Feb 1; 32(2): 118–26.
38. Ter-Pogossian MM et al. A positron-emission transaxial tomograph for nuclear imaging (PETT). Radiology 1975; 114(1): 89–98.
39. Hoffmann EJ, Phelps ME. Mullani NA, Higgins CS, Ter-Pogossian MM. Design and performance characteristics of a whole-body positron transaxial tomograph. J Nucl Med. 1976 Jun; 17(6): 493–502.
40. Raichle ME, Grubb RL, Gado MH, Eichling JO, Ter-Pogossiam MM. Correlation between regional cerebral blood flow and oxidative mechanism: In vivo studies in man. Arch Neurol. 1976 Aug; 33(8): 523–26.
41. Marcus E. Raichle, MD, interviewed by Sidney Goldring, MD. In: YouTube [Internet]. [cited 2020 Apr 20]. Available from: www.youtube.com/watch?v=XsDIpyaumIo.

9. THUNDERCLAP

1. Emilia Clarke. A Battle for My Life. In: The New Yorker [Internet]. [cited 2021 Apr 28]. Available from: https://www.newyorker.com/culture/personal-history/emilia-clarke-a-battle-for-my-life-brain-aneurysm-surgery-game-of-thrones.

REFERENCES

2. Milinis K, Thapar A, Neill K, Davies AH. History of Aneurysmal Spontaneous Subarachnoid Hemorrhage. Stroke. 2017 Oct; 48(10): e280–83.
3. Pool LJ. The Development of Modern Intracranial Aneurysm Surgery. Neurosurgery. 1977 Nov 1; 1(3): 233–37.
4. Del Maestro R. Harvey Cushing: A Life in Surgery. Can J Surg. 2007; 50(1): 70–71.
5. Doyle NM, Doyle JF, Walter EJ. The life and work of Harvey Cushing 1869–1939: A pioneer of neurosurgery. J Intensive Care Soc. 2017; 18(2): 157–58.
6. Wang H, Fraser K, Wang D, Lanzino G. The evolution of endovascular therapy for neurosurgical disease. Neurosurg Clin. 2005 Apr 1; 16(2): 223–29.
7. Mount LA. Results of treatment of intracranial aneurysms using the Selverstone clamp. J Neurosurg. 1959 Nov; 16: 611–18.
8. Moore CH, Murchison C. On a new method of procuring the consolidation of Fibrin in certain incurable Aneurisms. Medico-Chir Trans. 1864; 47: 129–49.
9. Guglielmi G. History of Endovascular Endosaccular Occlusion of Brain Aneurysms: 1965-1990. Interv Neuroradiol. 2007 Sep; 13(3): 217.
10. Pierot L, Wakhloo AK. Endovascular treatment of intracranial aneurysms: current status. Stroke. 2013 Jul; 44(7): 2046–54.
11. Aneurysm embolization: coiling, stenting, flow diversion. In: Mayfield Brain & Spine [Internet]. [cited 2019 Jan 8]. Available from: https://mayfieldclinic.com/pe-coiling.htm.

10. 'TIME IS BRAIN'

1. Goldstein M. Decade of the brain. An agenda for the nineties. West J Med. 1994 Sep; 161(3): 239–41.
2. Jones EG, Mendell LM. Assessing the Decade of the Brain. In: Science [Internet]. 1999 Apr 30 [cited 2022 Jan 26]. Available from: https://www.science.org/doi/abs/10.1126/science.284.5415.739.
3. Decade of the Brain. In: Wikipedia [Internet]. 2021 [cited 2022 Jan 26]. Available from: https://en.wikipedia.org/w/index.php?title=Decade_of_the_Brain&oldid=1036767112.
4. Gomez CR. Editorial: Time is brain! J Stroke Cerebrovasc Dis. 1993; 3(1): 1–2.
5. Basic Life Support (BLS). In: cpr.heart.org [Internet]. [cited 2022 May 9]. Available from: https://cpr.heart.org/en/cpr-courses-and-kits/healthcare-professional/basic-life-support-bls-training.
6. The History of ACLS Certification by American Heart Association. In: ACLS EDU [Internet]. 2018 [cited 2022 May 9]. Available from: https://aclsedu.com/the-history-of-acls-certification-by-american-heart-association/.
7. Advanced Cardiovascular Life Support (ACLS). In: cpr.heart.org [Internet]. [cited 2022 May 9]. Available from: https://cpr.heart.org/en/cpr-courses-and-kits/healthcare-professional/acls.
8. FAST (stroke). In: Wikipedia [Internet]. 2021 [cited 2022 May 9]. Available from: https://en.wikipedia.org/w/index.php?title=FAST_(stroke)&oldid=1023885094.
9. Caplan L. Introduction and perspective. In: Caplan L, editor. Caplan's Stroke: A Clinical Approach. Cambridge: Cambridge University Press; 2016. 1–18.

10. How do stroke units improve patient outcomes? A collaborative systematic review of the randomized trials. Stroke Unit Trialists Collaboration. Stroke. 1997 Nov; 28(11): 2139–144.
11. Alberts MJ, Hademenos G, Latchaw RE, Jagoda A, Marler JR, Mayberg MR, et al. Recommendations for the establishment of primary stroke centers. Brain Attack Coalition. JAMA. 2000 Jun 21; 283(23): 3102–109.
12. Alberts MJ, Wechsler LR, Jensen ME, Latchaw RE, Crocco TJ, George MG, et al. Formation and function of acute stroke-ready hospitals within a stroke system of care recommendations from the Brain Attack Coalition. Stroke. 2013 Dec 1; 44(12): 3382–393.
13. Towner J, Pieters T, Schmidt T, Pilcher W, Bhalla T. A History of Mobile Stroke Units and Review of Literature. Am J Interv Radiol 2018; 2(9): 1–5.

11. ABILITIES VERSUS DISABILITIES

1. Lanska DJ. The Historical Origins of Stroke Rehabilitation. In: Stein J, Harvey RL, Macko RF, Winstein CJ, Zorowitz RD, editors. Stroke Recovery and Rehabilitation. New York: Demos Medical Publishing; 2009. 3–30.
2. Rusk HA. A World to Care for: The Autobiography of Howard A. Rusk, M.D. New York: Random House; 1972. 328 p.
3. Taub E. Foreword for neuroplasticity and neurorehabilitation. In: Front Hum Neurosci [Internet]. 2014 Jul 24 [cited 2019 Feb 9]; 8. Available from: https://www.ncbi.nlm.nih.gov/pmc/articles/PMC4109562/.

4. Doidge N. The Brain That Changes Itself: Stories of Personal Triumph from the Frontiers of Brain Science. United Kingdom: Penguin; 2008. 533 p.
5. Edward Taub. In: Wikipedia [Internet]. 2018 [cited 2019 Feb 15]. https://en.wikipedia.org/w/index.php?title=Edward_Taub&oldid=85886212.
6. Over the Horizon. The Brain That Changes Itself - Full documentary. In: Youtube [Internet]. [cited 2019 Jan 18]. Available from: https://www.youtube.com/watch?v=bFCOm1P_cQQ.
7. Taub E, Uswatte G. Constraint-induced movement therapy: bridging from the primate laboratory to the stroke rehabilitation laboratory. J Rehabil Med. 2003 May; (41 Suppl): 34–40.
8. Kwakkel G, Veerbeek JM, van Wegen EEH, Wolf SL. Constraint-Induced Movement Therapy after Stroke. Lancet Neurol. 2015 Feb; 14(2): 224–34.
9. Wolf SL, Lecraw DE, Barton LA, Jann BB. Forced use of hemiplegic upper extremities to reverse the effect of learned non-use among chronic stroke and head-injured patients. Exp Neurol. 1989; 104: 125–32.
10. Wolf SL, Winstein CJ, Miller JP, et al. Effect of constraint-induced movement therapy on upper extremity function 3 to 9 months after stroke: the EXCITE randomized clinical trial. JAMA. 2006; 296(17): 2095–2104.
11. Silver Spring monkeys. In: Wikipedia [Internet]. 2019 [cited 2019 Feb 15]. Available from: https://en.wikipedia.org/w/index.php?title=Silver_Spring_monkeys&oldid=880337663.
12. NJTV News. Mirror Therapy Helps Patients Reduce Pain, Gain Mobility in Limbs. In: YouTube [Internet]. [cited 2019 Feb 25]. Available from: https://www.youtube.com/watch?v=1_KhO44mMq4.

REFERENCES

13. Ramachandran VS, Altschuler EL. The use of visual feedback, in particular mirror visual feedback, in restoring brain function. Brain. 2009 Jul 1; 132(7): 1693–710.
14. Tosi G, Romano D, Maravita A. Mirror Box Training in Hemiplegic Stroke Patients Affects Body Representation. In: Front Hum Neurosci [Internet]. 2018 Jan 4 [cited 2019 Feb 25]; 11. Available from: https://www.ncbi.nlm.nih.gov/pmc/articles/PMC5758498/.
15. Mirror Box Therapy/Mirror Visual Feedback. In: Research & Hope [Internet]. [cited 2019 Feb 25]. Available from: http://researchandhope.com/mirror-box-therapy-mirror-visual-feedback/.
16. Mirror box. In: Wikipedia [Internet]. 2019 [cited 2019 Feb 25]. Available from: https://en.wikipedia.org/w/index.php?title=Mirror_box&oldid=884415677.
17. Cortical homunculus. In: Wikipedia [Internet]. 2018 [cited 2019 Feb 15]. Available from: https://en.wikipedia.org/w/index.php?title=Cortical_homunculus&oldid=850542663.
18. Science in Seconds. Science in Seconds - Split Brain Syndrome. In: YouTube [Internet]. [cited 2019 Feb 16]. Available from: https://www.youtube.com/watch?v=u9u6cQYcOHw.
19. Norton A, Zipse L, Marchina S, Schlaug G. Melodic Intonation Therapy: Shared Insights on How it is Done and Why it Might Help. Ann N Y Acad Sci. 2009 Jul; 1169: 431–36.
20. Melodic Intonation Therapy. In: Research & Hope [Internet]. [cited 2019 Feb 16]. Available from: http://researchandhope.com/melodic-intonation-therapy/.
21. Tamplin J, Baker FA, Jones B, Way A, Lee S. "Stroke a Chord": the effect of singing in a community choir on mood and social engagement for people living with aphasia following a stroke.

NeuroRehabilitation. 2013; 32(4): 929–41. Available from: https://pubmed.ncbi.nlm.nih.gov/23867418/.
22. Claflin ES, Krishnan C, Khot SP. Emerging Treatments for Motor Rehabilitation After Stroke. Neurohospitalist. 2015 Apr; 5(2): 77–88.
23. Boonzaier J, van Tilborg GAF, Neggers SFW, Dijkhuizen RM. Noninvasive Brain Stimulation to Enhance Functional Recovery After Stroke: Studies in Animal Models. Neurorehabil Neural Repair. 2018 Nov; 32(11): 927–40
24. Cramer SC, Caplan LR. Chapter 20: Recovery, rehabilitation and repair. In: Caplan L, editor. Caplan's Stroke: A Clinical Approach. Cambridge: Cambridge University Press; 2016. 608–26.

12. STROKE IN THE YOUNG

1. Michael Rivkin, MD. In: Boston Children's Hospital [Internet]. [cited 2021 Jun 23]. Available from: https://www.childrenshospital.org/directory/physicians/r/michael-rivkin.
2. Stroke and Cerebrovascular Center. In: Boston Children's Hospital [Internet]. [cited 2021 Jun 23]. Available from: https://www.childrenshospital.org/centers-and-services/programs/o-_-z/cerebrovascular-disorders-and-stroke-program.
3. Department of Neurology. Our History. In: Boston Children's Hospital [Internet]. [cited 2021 Jun 23]. Available from: https://www.childrenshospital.org/centers-and-services/departments/neurology/meet-our-team/our-history.
4. Boston Children's Hospital. In: Wikipedia [Internet]. [cited 2021 Jun 23]. Available from: https://en.wikipedia.org/wiki/Boston_Children%27s_Hospital.

5. Boston Children's Hospital. History. In: Boston Children's Hospital [Internet]. [cited 2021 Jun 23]. Available from: https://bcrp.childrenshospital.org/history/boston-childrens-hospital/.
6. History. In: Boston Children's Hospital [Internet]. [cited 2021 Jun 23]. Available from: https://www.childrenshospital.org/research/about-us/history-link.
7. Ferriero DM, Fullerton HJ, Bernard TJ, Billinghurst L, Daniels SR, DeBaun MR, et al. Management of Stroke in Neonates and Children: A Scientific Statement From the American Heart Association/American Stroke Association. Stroke. 2019 Mar 1; 50(3): e51–96.
8. Caplan LR. Navigating the Complexities of Stroke. (Brain and Life Books). Oxford, New York: Oxford University Press; 2013. 288 p.

13. GENES

1. Chabriat H, Joutel A, Tournier-Lasserve E, Bousser MG. CADASIL: Yesterday, today, tomorrow. Eur J Neurol. 2020 Aug; 27(8): 1588–595.
2. The Discovery of CADASIL. In: Brain Facts [Internet]. [cited 2021 Aug 14]. Available from: https://www.brainfacts.org/Diseases-and-Disorders/Injury/2019/The-Discovery-of-CADASIL-040319.
3. Chabriat H, Joutel A, Dichgans M, Tournier-Lasserve E, Bousser MG. Cadasil. Lancet Neurol. 2009 Jul; 8(7): 643–53.
4. Fukutake T. Cerebral autosomal recessive arteriopathy with subcortical infarcts and leukoencephalopathy (CARASIL): From discovery to gene identification. J Stroke Cerebrovasc Dis. 2011 Apr; 20(2): 85–93.

5. Sickle Cell Disease. In: NHLBI, NIH [Internet]. [cited 2021 Jun 23]. Available from: https://www.nhlbi.nih.gov/health-topics/sickle-cell-disease.
6. Sickle cell disease. In: Wikipedia [Internet]. [cited 2021 Jun 23]Available from: https://en.wikipedia.org/wiki/Sickle_cell_disease.
7. Serjeant GR. One hundred years of sickle cell disease. Br J Hematol. 2010 Dec; 151(5): 425–29.
8. Linus Pauling. In: Wikipedia [Internet]. [cited 2021 Jun 23]. Available from: https://en.wikipedia.org/wiki/Linus_Pauling#Biological_molecules.
9. Vernon Ingram. In: Wikipedia [Internet]. [cited 2021 Jun 23]. Available from: https://en.wikipedia.org/w/index.php?title=Vernon_Ingram&oldid=1038204705.
10. Debette S, Caplan L. Genetics of stroke. In: Caplan L, editor. Caplan's Stroke: A Clinical Approach. Cambridge: Cambridge University Press; 2016. 129–44.
11. Candidate gene. In: Wikipedia [Internet]. 2021 [cited 2021 Aug 17]. Available from: https://en.wikipedia.org/w/index.php?title=Candidate_gene&oldid=1026115546.
12. Jonathan Rosand, MD. In: International Stroke Genetics Consortium [Internet]. [cited 2021 Aug 17]. Available from: www.strokegenetics.org/node/372.
13. What is the ISGC? In: International Stroke Genetics Consortium [Internet]. [cited 2021 Aug 17]. Available from: www.strokegenetics.org/what_is_isgc.
14. Raffeld MR, Debetter S, Woo D. International Stroke Genetics Consortium Update. Stroke. 2016 Apr 1; 47(4): 1144–145.

14. PREVENTION IS BETTER THAN CURE

1. Caplan L, Gorelick P. Stroke prevention. In: Caplan L, editor. Caplan's Stroke: A Clinical Approach. Cambridge: Cambridge University Press; 2016. 567–93.
2. Caplan LR. Navigating the Complexities of Stroke. (Brain and Life Books). Oxford, New York: Oxford University Press; 2013. 288 p.
3. Tattersall R. Diabetes: The Biography. Oxford: Oxford University Press; 2009.
4. History of Maggi in India. In: Transfin [Internet]. [cited 2021 Apr 10]. Available from: https://transfin.in/history-of-maggi-in-india.
5. Ruchika Shah. How much did Maggi ban cost Nestle India? In: DNA India [Internet]. [cited 2021 Apr 10]. Available from: https://www.dnaindia.com/business/report-how-much-did-maggi-ban-cost-nestle-india-2140196.
6. What's In a Cigarette? In: American Lung Association [Internet]. [cited 2021 Apr 10]. Available from: https://www.lung.org/quit-smoking/smoking-facts/whats-in-a-cigarette.
7. Shah RS, Cole JW. Smoking and stroke: the more you smoke the more you stroke. Expert Rev Cardiovasc Ther. 2010 Jul; 8(7): 917–32.
8. Benowitz NL. Nicotine Addiction. N Engl J Med. 2010 Jun 17; 362(24): 2295–303.
9. Maisch B. Alcoholic cardiomyopathy: The result of dosage and individual predisposition. Herz. 2016; 41(6): 484–93.
10. Aggarwal A, Pandian JD. Internet Gaming Disorder in undergraduate medical and dentistry students. CHRISMED J Health Res. 2019; 6: 237–41.

15. WORLD HISTORY AND STROKE

1. About Three Old Men: An Inquiry Into How Cerebral Arteriosclerosis Has Altered World Politics. In: Stroke [Internet]. [cited 2018 Dec 18]. Available from: https://www.ahajournals.org/doi/abs/10.1161/01.str.3.4.467.
2. dickmorrisreports. Woodrow Wilson, Mentally Impaired But Continued To Serve As President! In: Dick Morris TV: Lunch ALERT! [Internet]. YouTube. [cited 2018 Dec 18]. Available from: https://www.youtube.com/watch?v=LHMN7rL8q88.
3. Editors. Wilson embarks on tour to promote League of Nations. In: History [Internet]. [cited 2018 Dec 18]. Available from: https://www.history.com/this-day-in-history/wilson-embarks-on-tour-to-promote-league-of-nations.
4. Political Toast. American Presidents - Woodrow Wilson 28th US President. In: YouTube [Internet]. [cited 2018 Dec 18]. Available from: https://www.youtube.com/watch?v=2wsrF6SsI0U.
5. Striner R. The Surprising Evidence that Woodrow Wilson Was Suffering from a Brain Malfunction Before the Stroke that Crippled Him. In: History News Network [Internet]. [cited 2018 Jan 29]. Available from: http://historynewsnetwork.org/article/155787.
6. When a secret president ran the country. In: PBS NewsHour [Internet]. 2015 [cited 2018 Jan 29]. Available from: https://www.pbs.org/newshour/health/woodrow-wilson-stroke.
7. Ali R, Connolly ID, Li A, Choudhri OA, Pendharkar AV, Steinberg GK. The strokes that killed Churchill, Roosevelt, and Stalin. Neurosurgical Focus. 2016 Jul 1; 41(1): e7.
8. Stroke and the American presidency. In: PubMed [Internet]. [cited 2021 Jan 8]. Available from: https://pubmed.ncbi.nlm.nih.gov/17894986/.

9. Profiles of Aphasia: Dwight D. Eisenhower. In: National Aphasia Association [Internet]. 2017 [cited 2021 Jan 8]. Available from: https://www.aphasia.org/stories/aphasia-eisenhower/.
10. Loyola Medicine. Ten U.S. Presidents have Suffered Strokes. In: News Wise [Internet]. [cited 2021 Jan 8]. Available from: https://www.newswise.com/coronavirus/ten-u-s-presidents-have-suffered-strokes.
11. Famous People who Died of a Stroke. In: On This Day [Internet]. [cited 2021 Jan 8]. Available from: https://www.onthisday.com/people/cause-of-death/stroke#google_vignette.
12. Margaret Thatcher. In: On This Day [Internet]. [cited 2021 Jan 8]. Available from: https://www.onthisday.com/people/margaret-thatcher.
13. Yasser Arafat. In: On This Day [Internet]. [cited 2021 Jan 8]. Available from: https://www.onthisday.com/people/yasser-arafat.
14. John A. Macdonald. In: On This Day [Internet]. [cited 2021 Jan 8]. Available from: https://www.onthisday.com/people/john-a-macdonald.
15. Alexander Mackenzie. In: On This Day [Internet]. [cited 2021 Jan 8]. Available from: https://www.onthisday.com/people/alexander-mackenzie.
16. Catherine the Great. In: On This Day [Internet]. [cited 2021 Jan 8]. Available from: https://www.onthisday.com/people/catherine-the-great.
17. Isambard Kingdom Brunel. In: On This Day [Internet]. [cited 2021 Jan 8]. Available from: https://www.onthisday.com/people/isambard-kingdom-brunel.
18. Samuel de Champlain. In: On This Day [Internet]. [cited 2021 Jan 8]. Available from: https://www.onthisday.com/people/samuel-de-champlain.

19. Shirley Chisholm. In: On This Day [Internet]. [cited 2021 Jan 8]. Available from: https://www.onthisday.com/people/shirley-chisholm.
20. Ariel Sharon. In: Wikipedia [Internet]. 2020 [cited 2021 Jan 8]. Available from: https://en.wikipedia.org/w/index.php?title=Ariel_Sharon&oldid=995418061.
21. Atal Bihari Vajpayee. In: Wikipedia [Internet]. 2020 [cited 2021 Jan 8]. Available from: https://en.wikipedia.org/w/index.php?title=Atal_Bihari_Vajpayee&oldid=996555661.
22. Alexander von Humboldt. In: On This Day [Internet]. [cited 2021 Jan 9]. Available from: https://www.onthisday.com/people/alexander-von-humboldt.
23. John Logie Baird. In: On This Day [Internet]. [cited 2021 Jan 9]. Available from: https://www.onthisday.com/people/john-logie-baird.
24. Dorothy Hodgkin. In: On This Day [Internet]. [cited 2021 Jan 9]. Available from: https://www.onthisday.com/people/dorothy-hodgkin.
25. Watts S. The People's Tycoon: Henry Ford and the American Century. Random House, Inc.; 2006. In: Google Books [Internet]. Available from: https://books.google.com/books?id=LIDyU91YMHAC.
26. Gregory A. William Harvey, English physician. In: Encyclopædia Britannica [Internet]. Available from: https://www.britannica.com/biography/William-Harvey.
27. Marcello Malpighi. In: Wikipedia [Internet]. 2020 [cited 2021 Jan 9]. Available from: https://en.wikipedia.org/w/index.php?title=Marcello_Malpighi&oldid=996719034.
28. Edward Jenner. In: On This Day [Internet]. [cited 2021 Jan 9]. Available from: https://www.onthisday.com/people/edward-jenner.

29. Louis Pasteur. In: On This Day [Internet]. [cited 2021 Jan 9]. Available from: https://www.onthisday.com/people/louis-pasteur.
30. Elizabeth Blackwell. In: On This Day [Internet]. [cited 2021 Jan 9]. Available from: https://www.onthisday.com/people/elizabeth-blackwell.
31. Daniel Williams. In: On This Day [Internet]. [cited 2021 Jan 9]. Available from: https://www.onthisday.com/people/daniel-williams.
32. Gilman S, De Jong RN, 1907–1990. Ann of Neurology. 1991; 29(1): 108–09.
33. Hauw JJ. In memoriam: Dr. Raymond Escourolle (1924–1984). Acta Neuropathol. 1984 Jun 1; 65(2): 89.
34. Neurologist H. Houston Merritt is dead. JAMA. 1979 Feb 23; 241(8): 784.
35. Jill Bolte Taylor. In: Wikipedia [Internet]. 2021 [cited 2021 Jan 9]. Available from: https://en.wikipedia.org/w/index.php?title=Jill_Bolte_Taylor&oldid=998568807.
36. Charles Dickens. In: On This Day [Internet]. [cited 2021 Jan 9]. Available from: https://www.onthisday.com/people/charles-dickens.
37. Anne Morrow Lindbergh. In: On This Day [Internet]. [cited 2021 Jan 9]. Available from: https://www.onthisday.com/people/anne-morrow-lindbergh.
38. Bram Stoker. In: On This Day [Internet]. [cited 2021 Jan 9]. Available from: https://www.onthisday.com/people/bram-stoker.
39. Louisa May Alcott. In: On This Day [Internet]. [cited 2021 Jan 9]. Available from: https://www.onthisday.com/people/louisa-may-alcott.

40. Edith Wharton. In: On This Day [Internet]. [cited 2021 Jan 9]. Available from: https://www.onthisday.com/people/edith-wharton.
41. Charlie Chaplin. In: On This Day [Internet]. [cited 2021 Jan 9]. Available from: https://www.onthisday.com/people/charlie-chaplin.
42. Grace Kelly. In: On This Day [Internet]. [cited 2021 Jan 9]. Available from: https://www.onthisday.com/people/grace-kelly.
43. Luke Perry. In: On This Day [Internet]. [cited 2021 Jan 9]. Available from: https://www.onthisday.com/people/luke-perry.
44. Johann Sebastian Bach. In: Wikipedia [Internet]. 2021 [cited 2021 Jan 9]. Available from: https://en.wikipedia.org/w/index.php?title=Johann_Sebastian_Bach&oldid=998372010.
45. Felix Mendelssohn. In: On This Day [Internet]. [cited 2021 Jan 10]. Available from: https://www.onthisday.com/people/felix-mendelssohn.
46. Giuseppe Verdi. In: On This Day [Internet]. [cited 2021 Jan 10]. Available from: https://www.onthisday.com/people/giuseppe-verdi.
47. Sergei Prokofiev. In: Wikipedia [Internet]. 2021 [cited 2021 Jan 10]. Available from: https://en.wikipedia.org/w/index.php?title=Sergei_Prokofiev&oldid=999020472.
48. Wilson, Edith Bolling. My Memoir. Indianapolis: The Bobbs-Merrill Company, 1939.

Index

Abernethy, John, 52
acetylsalicylic acid or ASA, as aspirin, 67
ACLS certification, 129
acute chest syndrome, 168
Acute Stroke Ready Hospital (ASRH), 133
Adams, John Quincy, 191
Adams, Raymond D., 48, 50
Adler, Alfred, 30
advanced cardiac life support (ACLS), 128–29
alcohol, 174, 183–84; for preservation, 7
alcoholic cardiomyopathy, 184
Alcott, Louisa May, 196
alpha 2-antiplasmin, 78
Amarenco, Pierre, 45
Ambrose, James, 96
American Heart Association (AHA), 42, 45, 128–29
American Physiological Society, 58
Amphetamines, 162
anaesthesia, 53, 143, 158
anastomosis, 7, 50
anatomy, xvi, 2–3, 9–10, 12, 14, 23
Anderson, Carl, 107
aneurysm, 31, 52, 88, 112–24, 181–82; rupture, 115; saccular, 31, 122; types of (figure), 113
aneurysmal coiling, 84
Anhedonia, 183
Anichkov, Nikolai, 43
animal dissection, UGC banning, 17

235

Animal Liberation, Singer, 139
antibiotics, 72–73, 135
antihypertensive agents, 33
antiplatelets, 55
aorta (largest artery), xix–xx, 16, 55, 103
aorta, branches of (image), xx
'apoplexy,' xv–xvii, 8, 28, 32
apoplexy, reclassification on, 28
Arafat, Yasser, 192–93
Archimedes, 71
arterial vasodilation, 19
arteries: anterior cerebral, xx, xxi, 28; basilar, xx–xxi; brain, xix, 122, 161; cerebral hemispheres, xx; Circle of Willis, xxii; innominate, xix; left subclavian, xx; left vertebral, xx; metabolic control mechanism in, 18; middle cerebral, xx; neck, xix; posterior cerebral, xx–xxii, 160; right common carotid, xix; on right side of neck (image), xxi; right subclavian, xix; right vertebral, xix–xx, 8; supplying the brain (image), xxi; vertebral, 8, 28, 161
arteriopathies, 158–59, 161
arteriosclerosis, 37, 43
Arthur, Chester, 191–92

artificial breaths, 128
artificial radioisotopes, 109
aspirin, 56, 65–70, 72
aspirin prophylaxis, 70
Astrup, Tage, 77
atherosclerosis, 43–44, 47, 159, 162, 169, 174, 184
atrial fibrillation, 34, 37, 42, 50–51, 61, 65, 169, 182, 185
attention deficit hyperactivity disorder (ADHD), 186
auricles, 15
AutoCITE, 143
automated external defibrillator (AED), 128
autopsies, 11, 23–25, 27, 30, 40, 48–50, 70, 76, 86, 121, 142
Avenzoar, 23
Avery, Oswald T., 106
Avicenna, 23

Babinski, Joseph, 89, 91
Bach, Johann Sebastian, 197
bacterial: endocarditis, 159, 163; infections, 73
Baird, John Logie, 194
Banting, Fredrick G., 61, 106
basic life support (BLS), 128–29
Baskoff, 59

INDEX

Bayer, 67–68
Beatles, 94
BE-FAST, 131
Bell's palsy, 158
Benivieni, Antonio, 23
Best, Charles H., 61, 106
beta blockers, 33
Binswanger's disease, 164
black bile, xvi
Black, James, 33
Blackwell, Elizabeth, 195
bleeding, xvi, xviii, 51–52, 55–56, 62–64, 69, 73, 75, 77, 87, 127, 157–58, 162; in brain, xviii, 30; for vigour, 13
blindness, 49–50
Bloch, Felix, 98
Bloch, Konrad, 45
Block, Lawrence, 55
blood, xvi, 8–9, 18, 28, 73–74, 87–88, 95, 114, 126–27, 177; arterial, 13, 16, 159; 'circular' motion, 15; clot, xviii, 26–27, 34, 47, 55–56, 58, 75, 163, 182; deoxygenated, 31; haematoma, xix; oxygenation of, 128; types of, 13; venous, 13, 159
blood flow, circular motion, 13; diminished, xviii
bloodletting, 12–13, 32
blood lipids, abnormalities of, 177–78
blood pressure, 18, 32–33, 35, 118, 157, 175, 182; high, xviii, 30, 41, 127, 162, 174, 176; low, xviii
blood supply, xvii–xviii, 18, 54, 119, 126–128; abnormality in, xvii
blood thinners, 55, 127; types of, 35
blood vessels, 7, 10, 17, 28, 31, 82–83, 87–88, 90, 120, 122, 153, 160–63, 166–68, 174, 181–82; of brain, 158; rupture of small, xviii
BLS/ACLS, 128–30
Boston Children's Hospital (BCH), 151–55
Bouchard, Charles-Joseph, 31
Bousser, Marie-Germaine, 164–166
Bowes cell line, 79–80
Bowler, 166
Boyer, Herb, 80
Boyle, Robert, 5, 7
Boyle's Law, 7
brachiocephalic trunk, xix
brain: autopsies, 31; blood flow within, 19; Broca's area, 142, 146; capillaries, 19; cells, 19;

cortical homunculus, 142; dissection, 7; embolism, 50–51; haemorrhages, 83, 156, 158, 162, 183; infarcts, 159; injury, xvii, 117, 125; membranes around, 112; scans, 87, 117; vasculature, 7
Brain Attack Coalition (BAC), 132
Branting, Hjalmar, 187
'bridge therapy,' 61
Bright, Richard, 11
Brink, R.A., 62
Broca, Paul, 142
Brownell, Gordon, 109
Brown, Francis Henry, 151
Brown, Michael, 45
Brunel, Isambard Kingdom, 193
Buchner, Johann Andreas, 66
Budinger, Tom, 104
Busch, Christian, 71
Bush, George, 'Decade of the Brain' declaration, 125

Cadasil and Carasil, 164–67
cadavers, xvi, 9–10, 90
Caesar, Julius, invasion of Alexandria, 1
cancers, 70, 72, 78, 94, 100, 110, 153, 163, 173, 179, 181–82

The Canon of Medicine, Avenzoar, 23
capillaries, 16, 36, 165, 194
Caplan, Louis R., 50, 178
carbon dioxide, 19
cardiovascular diseases, 40, 128–129
cardiovascular system, 17
caregivers, 131, 150
Carlson, Peter, 141
carotid artery, xix–xxi, 2, 7–8, 28, 46–54, 90–91, 122, 159–61, 188; aneurysms, 118, 120; disease, 47, 49, 54; dissection, 51; endarterectomy, 51–54; ligation, 119–21; occlusion, 119; stenting, 54
Carpenter, Jeffery, 112
Carrea, Raúl, 52
Carswell, Robert, 11
Casserio, Giulio, 5
Catherine the Great, 193
catheter-based mechanical thrombectomy, 83
Cederlund, Jan, 38–39
cellulitis, 73
cephalin, 59–60
cerebral: aneurysms, 118–20, 123; angiography, 88–93; autosomal recessive arteriopathy, 166; blood

INDEX

flow (perfusion), 19;
embolism (clots in the
brain), 28; haemorrhage,
194; hemispheres, xx
Cerebri Anatome (*The Anatomy
of the Brain and Nerves*),
Willis, 7
Champlain, Samuel de, 193
Chaplin, Charlie, 196
Charcot, Jean-Martin, 31
Charcot–Bouchard aneurysms,
31
Chargaff, 61
Charles, Arthur F., 60
Charles I, 12, 14
Charles II, 12
chest compressions, 128
childhood brain ischemia, 159
childhood stroke, 156
child neurology, 154
Chisholm, Shirley, 193
cholesterol-lowering agents, 44
cholesterols, 42–44, 47, 159,
162, 177–78
Churchill, Winston, xv, 190;
death of, 190; image, 191
chyle, 2, 15
cigarettes, 174, 181; nicotine,
181–183
Circle of Willis, xxii, 1, 7–8,
123; image, xxii

Clarke, Emilia Isobel Euphemia
Rose, 112, 114–17, 196
cloning, 81–82
clots, 21, 27–28, 55, 73, 79,
82–83, 114, 121, 126–27,
162; formation, 34–35, 53,
56–57, 69, 74–75, 119,
161, 170, 185; lysis (break
down), 75, 77; retrieval
devices, 84
coagulation cascade, figure, 57
Cohen, Stanley, 80
Cohnheim, Julius, 28
Collen, Désiré, 78–79, 81
Collip, James B., 106
colour printing technique, *la
poupée*, 11
comprehensive stroke centre
(CSCs), 132–33
computed tomography
(CT), 48, 107, 110, 133;
angiograms, 87; scanner, 87,
96, 111, 133; scans, 86–87,
93–97, 126–27, 164
constraint-induced movement
therapy (CIMT), 139, 143
contrast-enhanced computed
tomography (CECT), 97
Cooley, Denton, 54
Cooper, Astley, Sir, 52, 118
Cope, Freeman Winder, 98

Cormack, Allan M., 93
coronary: angiography, 76; thrombosis, 76
corpus callosum, 146–47, 149
Corradi, Alfonso, 122
Craven, Lawrence L., 69
Crohn's disease, 163
Cruveilhier, Jean, 11
crystallography, 194
CT scans. *See* computed tomography (CT)
'cuorin,' 60
Curie, Marie, 38, 108
Curie, Pierre, 38
Cushing, Harvey, 118–20
cysticercosis, 163

Damadian, Raymond, 97–100, 102–03, 105–16
Dandy, Walter, 120
DeBakey, Michael, 53
De Humani Corporis Fabrica, 4, 24
De Humani Corporis Fabrica, Vesalius, 4
dehydration, xviii, 167, 186
DeJong, Russell, 195
Denier, André, 38
depression, 150
De Sedibus et Causis Morborum per Anatomen Indagatis (*The Seats and Causes of Diseases Investigated by Anatomy*), Morgagni, 24–25
De Usu Partium Corporis Humani (*On the Usefulness of the Parts of the Body*), 2
DeWood, Marcus, 76
diabetes, 48, 80, 159, 162, 169, 174–77, 183
diacetylmorphine, 68
Dickens, Charles, 196
digital resources, 10
digital subtraction angiogram (DSA), 88
digital subtraction angiography, 92–93
Dirac, Paul, 107
diuretic chlorothiazide, 33
Doidge, Norman, 134, 139
dopamine, 183
Doppler, Christian, 87
Doppler ultrasound, 87
Dott, Norman, 120
Dreser, Heinrich, 67–69
drugs, 21–22, 45, 55–56, 64–69, 72, 78, 80, 153, 162, 175, 178; anticoagulant, 35, 55–57, 60, 64; antihypertensive, 33; antiplatelet, 35, 56; clot-dissolving, 83, 126–27; illicit use, 162
Dussik, Friedrich, 38

Dussik, Karl Theodore, 38
dysarthria (difficulty speaking), 190

Ebers Papyrus, 65
echocardiogram, 31, 35, 40, 73
echocardiography, 38–40
Eclampsia, 162
E. coli, 80
Edison, Thomas A., 172
Edler, Inge, 38–40
Edwards, Mary, 52
Eichengrün, Arthur, 67–68
Einstein, Albert, 172
Einthoven, Willem, 37
Eisenhower, Dwight D., 64, 192
EKG machine, 102; see also echocardiogram
electrocardiogram ECG), 31, 35–38
electrocardiography, 37
electrolysis, 124
electrothrombosis or galvanopuncture, 122, 124
embalming, 9
embolism, 27, 47, 158–59
EMI Mark I, 95
Emmett Holt, 60
The Emperor of All Maladies, Mukherjee, 179
empyema (pus around the lungs), 75

encéphalographie artérielle (arterial encephalography), 90
Enders, John, 153
Endo, Akira, 45
endovascular treatment, 123
Erasistratus, 23
Erlandsen, 59
Escourolle, Raymond, 195
Ettinger, 184
'eukrasia,' xvi
European Society of Pathology, 26
executed criminals, 4, 10, 14
Exercitatio Anatomica de Motu Cordis et Sanguinis in Animalibus (On the Motion of the Heart and Blood), Harvey, 16–17
Experimental NMR Conference (ENC), Virginia, 104

Fabricius, Hieronymus, 14
Fabry disease, 159
Falloppio, Gabriele, 5
Farber, Sidney, 153
Fassbender, 133
'FAST,' 130, see also BE-FAST
fibrillation, 185
fibrinogen, 56, 58, 74–75
fibrinolysin (later streptokinase), 75

fibrinolysis, 78, 81
Fillmore, Millard, 191
Firestone, Floyd, 39
Fisher, Charles Miller, 47–50, 52
Fisher, Doris, 47
fleams, 12
Fleming, David, 52
Fogarty catheter, 77
Folkman, Judah, 153
FONAR, 103
Food Safety and Standards Authority of India (FSSAI), 180
Ford, Gerald, 192
Ford, Henry, 194
forensic medicine, 22, 29
formaldehyde (formalin), 9
Framingham Heart Study, 40–42, 44
Framingham Risk Score, 42
Freeman, Walter, 92, 98
Frei, 123
Friends of Framingham Heart Study, 41
Froriep, Robert, 25, 27
Fuller, Thomas, 172
Fulton, John, 20

Galen of Pergamon, xvi, 1–6, 12–13, 23
gallbladder, 18
Galvani, Luigi, 35
galvanometer, 35
Game of Thrones, 112, 114, 117
Garner, R.L., 75
Genentech, 80–81
General Magnetic, 104
genome-wide association studies (GWAS), 42, 170
Georgia Warm Springs Foundation, 135
glomerulus, 18
glucose, xvii, 19
Gofman, John, 44
Gohr, H., 38
Goldsmith, Michael, 71, 102–03
Goldstein, Joseph, 45
González-Crussi, Francisco, 92
Gortner, Ross A., 62
Grayson, 188–89
Gross, Robert E., 153
Gruentzig, Andreas, 93
Guglielmi, Guido, 124

Hachinski, 166
haemorrhage, xvi–xix, 30, 87, 121, 127, 147, 157; aneurysmal subarachnoid, 51; intracranial, 31–32; subarachnoid (SAH), 31, 114–15, 158

INDEX

haemorrhagic apoplexy/stroke, 28, 30–33, 55, 97, 127, 155–56, 160, 163, 182, 190
haemothorax (blood around the lungs), 75
Hall, John E., 153
Handbuch der Physiologie (Handbook of Physiology), Müller, 25
hand tapping, 148
Harvey, Eliab, 13
Harvey, William, 12–16, 194; death of, 17–21
Haywood, Carolyn, 151
heart, xviii–xix, 2, 13–16, 18–19, 35–39, 42, 60, 128, 158–59, 162, 174, 177, 184; chambers of, 30; emboli from, 34; left atrium, 30–31, 38–39; left ventricle, 15, 30–31, 38; rhythm, 35, 184; right ventricle, 30; transplant, 153; valves, 159, 163
heart (the pump), xviii–xix
heart attacks/failure, 29, 33–34, 42–45, 64, 69–70, 72–73, 81, 126, 128–30, 173–74, 182–83
heart disease, 30, 37, 40–42, 53, 128–29, 159, 162, 174, 177

Hebenstreit, 51
hemiplegia, 49, 51
'heparin,' 50, 53, 56–57, 60, 64; production, 61; as protamine sulphate, 61
'hepraphosphatide,' 60
heroin, 67–69, 162
Herophilus of Chalcedon, 1, 23
Herrick, James, 168
Hertz, Gustav, 39–40
Heyneker, Herb, 81
high cholesterol, 174, 177–78
high-density lipoprotein (HDL) (good) cholesterol, 42, 44, 177, 182
high-resolution computed tomography (HRCT), 97
Hilal, 124
Hill, Leonard, Sir, 20
Hippocrates, xv–xvi, 6, 23, 65; father of medicine, xv
Hippocratic, humours of, xvi
HIV/AIDS, 161, 163
Hodgkin, Dorothy, 194
Hoffman, 67–68
holiday heart syndrome, 184
Holt, 60
Hooper, Robert, 11
Horsley, Victor, 118
Hounsfield, Godfrey N., 93–96, 107, 111
Hounsfield scale, 96

Howell, William Henry, 57–60
human dissections, 1–2, 4
Humboldt, Alexander von, 193
humoral theory, xvi, 12
hydrogen ion, 19
hypertension, 30–33, 127, 159, 169, 174, 176, 182–83, 186; cuff-based sphygmomanometer, 32; or 'hard pulse disease,' 32; Korotkoff sounds, 32; reninangiotensin system, 33; salt restriction, 32; treatment of, 32
hypophysis (pituitary gland), 2

Ibn al-Nafis, 23
Ignatowski, A.I., 43
Iles, Thomas, 6
imaging, 86–88, 95, 99
infections, 73, 121, 158–61, 163, 167
Ingram, Vernon, 169
insulin, 61, 80–81, 106, 177; discovery of, 61, 106
International Normalized Ratio (INR), 65
International Stroke Genetics Consortium (ISGC), 170–71
International Subarachnoid Aneurysm Trial, 124

internet gaming disorder (IGD), 185
intestines, 10, 18
intracranial aneurysms, 122–23
intracranial pressure (ICP), 119
intravenous injection, 7
The Invisible College, as Philosophical College, 5, 7
ischemia, xvii–xviii, 87, 126; in children, 158
ischemic, 21, 32; penumbra, 127; strokes, 34–35, 72, 77, 82, 87, 126–27, 156, 159, 162, 182, 184–85
'ischemic' (Virchow's term) apoplexy, 28
Itano, Harvey, 168

James I, 14
Jenner, Edward, 194
John of Salisbury, xv
Johnson, Andrew, 191–92
Joliot-Curie, Iréne, 107–09
Joliot, Jean Frédéric, 108
Joslin, Elliott Proctor, 175–76

Kean, Sam, 164
Kelly, Grace, 196
Kenealy, Lori, 141
Kennedy, Rosemary, 92
kidneys, 18, 43, 98, 194
Kinsell, Laurence, 44

INDEX 245

Kolbe, Hermann, 66
Kölliker, Rudolf Albert von, 35
Koop, C. Everett, 183
Korotkoff, Nikolai, 32
Kreel, Louis, 96
Kuhl, David, 110

Lacerada, Ruy, 92
Ladd, William, 153
lancet, 12, 66
Lauterbur, Paul, 99–101, 103, 105
Lawrence, Ernest, 109
League of Nations, 187–90
learned paralysis, 144
Le Blon, Jacob Christoph, 11
Lederle Laboratories, 76
leeches, application of, 32
left ventricular hypertrophy, 31, 37
Lenin, Vladimir, 190
leucotomies, 91–92
'leukemia,' 26
leukoencephalopathy (CADASIL), 165–66
Lima, Almeida, 92
Lindbergh, Anne Morrow, 196
Link, Karl Paul Gerhard, 62
Lippmann, Gabriel, 36
liver, 2, 13, 15, 18, 44, 60, 157
Locke, John, 5

low-density lipoprotein (LDL), 44, 177, 182
Lower, Richard, 5, 7
Luessenhop, 122
lungs, 2, 18–19, 27, 31, 34, 96, 103, 182, 194; cancer, 179, 181–82
Lyme disease, 161
Lynen, Feodor, 45

Macdonald, John A., 193
Mackenzie, Alexander, 193
MacLagan, Thomas John, 66
Macleod, John J.R., 106
Maggi noodles, 180–81
magnetic resonance angiograms (MRA), 87, 156
magnetic resonance imaging (MRI), 21, 48, 87, 96–106, 111, 115, 126, 156, 158, 164–65; 'Mink 5,' 103
magnetic resonance venography (MRV), 156
malarial fever (ague), willow tree bark for, 66
Malpighi, Marcello, 16, 23, 194
Mansfield, Peter, 101, 103–05
Maryland's Prevention of Cruelty to Animals, 141
Massachusetts General Hospital (MGH), 50, 110, 170
Matteucci, Carlo, 35

Maudsley, Andrew, 101
McLean, Jay, 57–60
Mechanical Embolus Removal in Cerebral Ischemia (MERCI), 84–85
melodic intonation therapy, 147
Mendelssohn, Felix, 197
MERCI corkscrews, 85
MERCI retrievers, 84
Merritt, H. Houston, 195
Meschia, J., 191
METASTROKE consortium, 171
Meyer, John S., 77
microbiology, 22, 167
migraines, 115, 158–59, 161, 166, 185–86
Miller, Bill, 153
Miller Fisher syndrome, 51
Minkoff, Larry, 102–03
mirror therapy, 144
mitochondrial disorders, 159
mobile game, Candy Crush Saga, 185
Moniz, António Egas, 88–92, 105
monosodium glutamate (MSG), 180
Moore, Charles, 121
Moralez, Audrey, 71

Morgagni, Giovanni, 23–25
Morris, Peter, 103
Mosso, Angelo, 19
moyamoya disease, 159–60
MSUs (Mobile Stroke Unit), 133
Muirhead, Alexander, 35
Mukherjee, Siddhartha, 179
Müller, Heinrich, 35
Müller, Johannes Peter, 25
Müller, Paul Hermann, 106
Murchison, Charles, 121
myocardial infarction (MI), 73, 76–77
myocardial necrosis (heart muscle damage), 76

Nathan, David, 153
National Foundation for Infantile Paralysis, 135; 'President's Birthday Ball,' 136
National Institutes of Health (NIH), 100, 140–41, 143
'natural pneuma' or 'spirit,' 2
nervous system, xviii, 18, 134, 137
Nestlé, 180
neuro-anaesthesia, 120
neurology, 2, 50–51, 89, 97, 154, 170

INDEX

neurons, xviii, 19–20, 126–27, 134, 143, 149
neuroplasticity, 137–43, 147
neurosurgery, 97, 122, 154
neurotransmitters, 150, 183
Nixon, Richard M., 192
Nobel, Alfred, 105
Nobel Prize, 36, 39, 70, 91–92, 96, 105–06, 153
non-invasive brain stimulation, 148–49; transcranial magnetic stimulation (TMS), 149
non-invasive tests, 88
nuclear magnetic resonance (NMR), 98

O'Connor, Basil, 136
Olson, 61
oral contraceptive use, 186, *see also* drugs
organs, 7, 18, 20, 23, 48
Osler, William, Sir, 4, 119
oxygen, xvii, 17, 19, 54, 89, 160, 167, 182

Pacheco, Alex, 139–41
paediatrics, 151–52
paediatric stroke, 155
pancreas, 18
parasitology, 29

Paré, Ambroise, 46, 51
Pasteur, Louis, 172, 194–95
pathology, 2, 11, 20, 22, 26, 48, 136, 167; of contagion, 23; history of, 23; of stroke, 11
Pauling, Linus Carl, 168
Penfield, Wilder, 48
Pennica, Diane, 81
penumbra system, 83
People for the Ethical Treatment of Animals, or PETA, 139–41
perinatal stroke, 156
peripheral arteries, 31, 43, 88
Permin, Per M., 77
Perry, Luke, 196
PET SCAN, 107–11
Petty, William, Sir, 5
pharmacology, 2, 22, 167
Phelps, Michael, 111
phlegm, xvi
Physical Medicine and Rehabilitation (PM&R), 135
physiology, 2, 9, 12, 14, 20, 25, 37, 58–59
piezoelectricity, 38
Piria, Raffaele, 66
pituitary basophilia (Cushing syndrome), 119

plaque, 43, 47, 53, 56, 177–78
plasma, 74
plasmin, 75, 77–78
plasminogen, 75, 77
Platelet activation, 56
plexus, 2, 5
pneumoencephalography, 89
pneumonia, 18, 68
point-of-care laboratory equipment, 133
polio virus, 135–36, 153; vaccines against, 153; victims, 135, 152
polycythemia, 159
Porter, Roy, 4
positron emission tomography (PET), 21, 107, 110–11
positron emission transaxial tomography (PETT), 111
post-mortem examinations. *See* autopsies
primary stroke centre (PSCs), 132–33
printing techniques, 10
Prokofiev, Sergei, 197
protamine as salmine, 61
prothrombin time determinants, 65
pulmonary: angiography, 77; embolism, 28, 77; hypertension, 19

pulseless ventricular tachycardia, 128
Purcell, Edward, 98
Pykett, Ian, 103

Rabi, I., 98
Ramachandran, V.S., 134, 144
rats, Walker sarcoma tumours, 99
red blood cells, 56, 159–60, 167–69
refractory epilepsy, 146
Regan, 184
Rehabilitation for stroke victims, 136
Reinhardt, Benno Ernst Heinrich, 26
rete mirabile, 1–2, 4; tortuous structure of, 2; 'wonderful net,' 1
rheumatism, 68; salicin against, 67
Rifkin, Daniel B., 78
Rijken, Dingeman, 79
risk factors, 41–42, 44, 156, 159, 164, 166, 173–77, 184
Riva-Rocci, Scipione, 32
Rivkin, Michael, 154–55
Robbins, Frederick, 153
Robbins Textbook of Basic Pathology, Virchow, 22
Roberts, William C., 76

INDEX 249

Rokitansky, Carl, 25, 30, 42
Roosevelt, Franklin D., 32–33, 135, 190–92: death of, 32–33, 190; image, 191
Rosand, Jonathan, 170
Rotch, Thomas Morgan, and bacteria-free milk, 153
Royal Society of London, 5, 66
Roy, Charles Smart, 20
Rusk, Howard A., 125

Sabin, Albert Bruce, 153
Safirstein, B.E., 191
salicin, 66
salicylic acid, 66–68
Salk, Jonas, 153
Salk Vaccine Field Trial, 136
Saryan, Leon, 99
Schiller, Francis, xvii
Schmidt-Mulheim, 57
Schoeffel, Eugen Wilhem, 63
Schofield, Frank, 62
Scott, David A., 60
seizures, 158, 160
Seldinger, Sven Ivar, 92
Serbinenko, Fedor A., 123
serendipity, 71–72
The Serendipity Mindset, Busch, 71
serum, 74
SHARe project, 42
Sharon, Ariel, 193

Sherrington, Charles Scott, 20
Sherry, Sol, 75–76
A Short History of Medicine, González-Crussi, 92
Sicard, Jean-Athanase, 89, 91
sickle cell disease, 153, 159–60, 167–69
Silver, Spencer, 72
Singer, Peter, 139
Singer, S.J., 168
single photon emission computed tomography (SPECT), 110
skin disease, 23
skull, xviii–xx, 8, 46, 91, 97, 112, 114, 116, 143, 159–60
Smith, W.K., 62
smoking, 41, 159, 162, 179, 181–83, 186
somatostatin, 80–81
soporales, 46
Sperry Ultrasonic Reflectoscope, 39
'split-brain syndrome,' 146
Stalin, Joseph, 190–91; death of, 190; image, 191
statins, 45, 178, *see also* drugs
stent retrievers, 84–85
Stoker, Bram, 196
Stone, Edward, 66
streptococci, 73–75
streptokinase, 73–77

streptokinase preparation, 76
stroke, xvii; care, 72, 132;
    causes of, xix, 155, 158,
    161–62, 164; diagnoses, 86;
    divisions of, xvii; mimics,
    158; neurologists, 131; and
    world politics, 187–91
stroke patients, xvii, 35, 126,
    131–32, 139, 149–50;
    aspirin prevention clinical
    trials in, 165; cortical
    reorganization, 143
Stroke Prevention by Aggressive
    Reduction in Cholesterol
    Levels (SPARCL), 45
stroke units and Stroke Centres,
    131–33, 136
suction thrombectomy, 84
Sutures, 120
sweet clover, 62–63; coumarin
    in, 63; and cows' death, 62
sweet clover disease, 62, 64
Sweet, William, 109
synapses, 134
Synthetic insulin, 80
syphilis, 161, 163
systemic blood pressures, 19
systemic haemorrhage, 83

Taub, Edward, 137–41, 143;
    'learned non-use,' 144; Silver
Spring monkeys, 139–40,
    142
Taylor, Jill Bolte, 195
telemedicine capabilities, 133
Ter-Pogossian, Michel, 110–11
Tesla, Nikola, 86
*A Textbook of Physiology for
    Medical Students and
    Physicians*, Howell, 58
Thatcher, Margaret, 192
Theresa, Sister, 152
thoracic aortic aneurysm, 121
thrombectomies, 82–85, 132
thromboembolism, 64, 84, 161
thrombolytic therapy, 76–77
'The Thromboplastic Action of
    Cephalin,' McLean, 60
thrombosis, 27–28, 90, 119,
    122, 158, 163
thunderclap headache, 112,
    114, see also migraines
Tillett, William Smith, 74–75
'time is brain,' xviii, 125–26
tissue plasminogen activator
    (tPA), 75, 77
Todd's paresis, 158
tonsils, 69, 161
Tournier-Lasserve, Elisabeth,
    165–66
tPA (rtPA), tissue plasminogen
    activator, 73, 75, 77–79,
    81–83, 127, 133

INDEX

transcranial magnetic stimulation (TMS), 149
transient ischemic attacks (TIAs), 49–50, 56, 70, 178–79
trauma, 19, 156, 159, 161–62
tuberculosis, 63, 68, 163
'Tumour Detection by Nuclear Magnetic Resonance,' Damadian, 99
Tyler, John, 191–92
typhus epidemic, 26
Tzu, Sun, 112

Ultrasonic Reflectoscope, 39
urokinase (isolated from human urine), 77

Vajpayee, Atal Bihari, 193
Valsalva, 25
Vane, John, 70
Varicellazoster virus (VZV), 161
vascular: malformations, 20, 28, 88, 158; neurosurgery, 120; resistance, 17; structure, 1, 5, 7, 87
vasoconstriction, 17, 19
vasodilation, 17–18
veins, xix, 13, 15–16, 26, 28, 87, 156, 158–59, 162–63
Velasquez, 122

venous thrombosis, 156
ventricles, 4, 15, 34, 95
ventricular fibrillation, 128
ventriculography (pneumoencephalography), 91
Verdi, Giuseppe, 197
Vesalius, Andreas, 3–5, 10, 12, 14, 24, 119; medical career, 3; public dissection, 4
Vesling, Johann, 5
Vincent, Clovis, 91
Vinci, Leonardo da, 1
Virchow–Robin spaces, 28
Virchow, Rudolf Ludwig Carl, 22, 25–29
Virchows Archiv, 26
Virchow's node, 28
Virchow's Triad, 22, 27, 34, 161
virtual simulators, 10
'vitality,' xvi
vitamin K, 64, 157
vosospasm, 114

Waller, Augustus Desiré, 36–38
Wallis, John, 5
Walter K., 20
warfarin—'warf,' 56, 61–62, 64–65, 157, 192; as rat poison, 64
Wedekin, T.H., 38

Weimar, Willem, 79
Weiss, Harvey J., 70
Weller, Thomas, 153
Wells, Ibert, 168
Wepfer, Johann Jakob, xv, 5
Wharton, Edith, 196
Williams, Daniel, 195
Willis, Thomas, 5–7, 10
Wilson, Edith, 188
Wilson, Woodrow, 187–90, 192
Windaus, Adolf, 43
wine, and preservation of brain, 7, *see also* alcohol

World Instant Noodles Association, 180
World War II, 33, 135, 152, 190
Wren, Christopher, 5, 7–8
Wright, Charles Romley Alder, 68

X-rays, 86, 93

yellow bile, xv

zeugmatography, 100

About the Author

Dr Aishwarya Aggarwal was born in India to a family of doctors. Her father is a surgeon and her mother is a gynaecologist. She completed her medical training at Christian Medical College, Ludhiana, and is currently a neurology resident at John F. Kennedy Medical Center, New Jersey, USA. After completing the residency, she plans to pursue fellowships in vascular neurology and neurointerventional surgery.

Dr Aggarwal has previously co-authored an academic book, *Stories of Stroke*, with Dr Louis R. Caplan and several other prominent neurologists from across the globe. She has also authored many research papers. Outside of work, she enjoys playing badminton, photography and dancing.

HarperCollins *Publishers* India

At HarperCollins India, we believe in telling the best stories and finding the widest readership for our books in every format possible. We started publishing in 1992; a great deal has changed since then, but what has remained constant is the passion with which our authors write their books, the love with which readers receive them, and the sheer joy and excitement that we as publishers feel in being a part of the publishing process.

Over the years, we've had the pleasure of publishing some of the finest writing from the subcontinent and around the world, including several award-winning titles and some of the biggest bestsellers in India's publishing history. But nothing has meant more to us than the fact that millions of people have read the books we published, and that somewhere, a book of ours might have made a difference.

As we look to the future, we go back to that one word—a word which has been a driving force for us all these years.

Read.

    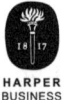 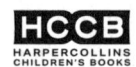

 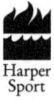